Social Issues

Social Issues

Edited by

Georgeta Rață and Patricia-Luciana Runcan

CAMBRIDGE
SCHOLARS
PUBLISHING

Social Issues,
Edited by Georgeta Raţă and Patricia-Luciana Runcan

This book first published 2014

Cambridge Scholars Publishing

12 Back Chapman Street, Newcastle upon Tyne, NE6 2XX, UK

British Library Cataloguing in Publication Data
A catalogue record for this book is available from the British Library

ISBN (10): 1-4438-5676-2, ISBN (13): 978-1-4438-5676-8

TABLE OF CONTENTS

Chapter Three: Vulnerable Populations

LIST OF TABLES

List of Illustrations

FOREWORD

This collection of essays gathers papers dealing with different social issues formally grouped under *Faces of Migration* and *Vulnerable Populations*. Though, in general, *social issues* are distinguished from *economic issues*, both migration and vulnerability have economic causes.

The first chapter presents the different faces of migration – both seen (Delia-Ioana Nadolu, Maria-Ana Georgescu and Emilia Herman, Florentin Vlad, and Beniamin Lup) and unseen (Ramona Malița), analysing the socio-economic causes and consequences of migration and, implicitly, of urban depopulation in Romania and of human trafficking approached from a double perspective (as a modern form of slavery and as an infringement of European Values).

The second chapter attempts at identifying the mechanisms used in social issue societies in the construction of identity, from a double perspective: diachronic (Daniela-Mihaela Spînu-Dumitru, Alin Gavreliuc and Dana Gavreliuc) and synchronic (Claudia-Anamaria Iov, Lavinia-Elisabeta Popp and Felicia Andrioni, Amador Jimenez-Garrido and Eufrasio Perez-Navio, Claudia-Livia Andrițoi, Marian Mihăilă, Ştefan-Sebastian Maftei, Ştefania Bejan, Dănuț-Ioan Craşovan and Delia Tomici, Maria Constantinescu and Cornel Constantinescu, and Dan-Ioan Dascălu). The elderly, the homeless, the immigrants, the minorities (the Roma) are scrutinised with emphasis on the network society, on the right to self-determination, on social integration, on trauma.

The third chapter focuses on personal issues rather than social issues. The essays deal with such issues as work-family conflict and couple's satisfaction with life (Delia Vîrgă, Silvia Rusu and Roxana Sârbu), problem behaviour in autistic children (Laura-Cristina Oprică), intestinal Giardiasis in institutionalized elderly patients (Iosif Marincu, Ioana Todor and Mihai Mareş), respiratory pathology in residents living close to lignite quarries (Delia Nica-Badea), chronic alcohol consumption in patients with liver disease (Elena Toader), and political persecution and extradition of criminals (Claudia-Livia Andrițoi and Adina-Iulia Nicolae).

The Editors

JANUS BIFRONS, OR THE UNSEEN FACE OF MIGRATION

RAMONA MALIȚA

Introduction

Francophone literature is a particular, special and provoking case in the concept of migration, involving other adjacent notions such as linguistic identity, bilingualism, expatriation, exodus, diaspora, etc. The multitude of (in)congruent purports shows the researcher various insights and triggers unforeseen, complex constellations, since the phenomenon itself—francophony—is full of meanderings that can be read not only from an aesthetic, ethic or moral point of view, but also from a political one. A visual reading of the francophone world map makes visible the extended geographical space of the seventy-eight countries acknowledged as operating under the aegis of the French language, from the Tropic of Cancer to the Tropic of Capricorn, passing through cultures, religions, climates, races of people, mentalities, customs, politically-coloured governments, different morals, being surprising, unequal and even opposed at times; in other words, it is odd and fragmentary. Nonetheless, for the informed eye this map represents the maze of a certain literary typology, characterised by strong personalities, specific themes and motifs, Nobel prizes for Literature, aesthetic paradigms that are canonical for the present literature, and, above all, the generous concept of humanitas. Our research focuses on the aesthetic literary illustration of four social concepts—transmigration, statelessness, multilingualism and bilingualism—in francophone literature. The devastating experiences that lead to the hurting/injuring and finally the loss of the inner identity, the social maladjustment or the mere refusal to adapt, and the compulsory belonging to a territory—the community of diaspora—that the family imposes on its immigrant members are the means by which we investigate the characters of some francophone novels using obvious and certified auctorial autobiographical insertions. This interdisciplinarity is based on the relation of (in)congruence between the biography of the author as an emigrant, the fiction of the text published in diaspora, the reception of the message in the reference community, the formation of an aesthetic and social horizon of expectations, and the creation of a public opinion.

Research Methods

The comparative analysis is the one through which we build relations of congruence, incongruence, inadvertence, convergence or divergence between novels dealing with the theme of migration on the francophone territory in general, and on the Arab land in particular. The novels we refer to are *Amours sauvages* by Calixthe Beyala,[1] *Ils disent que je suis une beurette* by Soraya Nini, and *Beur's story* by Ferrudja Kessas. **The thematic analysis** brings a special input in detecting forms, shades, surrogates, types, structures and literary *autobiographemes*, together with the social spreading of the phenomenon of migration. **The historical paraliterary analysis** explains, fathoms, sustains and exploits the literary fiction in the aforementioned novels.

Discussion

Non nova, sed nove. Our research, starting with a literary approach and announces some social phenomena of the present day, is an interrogative-ascertaining approach implying a triple vector: *Primo*: in which way do the social and the historical aspects influence the literary? *Secundo*: to what extent are the macro-historical elements present in the micro-history (in the concrete destinies of the characters/people)? *Tertio*: to what extent is literature received in a society prepared (or not) to accept and benefit from the presence of the immigrant with (or without) a legal residence? The specialists judge that the predominant themes of the francophone literature—the identity quest, the woman's status, the social opposition white vs. black people, social, racial, and sexual discrimination and interbreeding—are the parameters through which the destiny of the characters is drawn, whether they are main or secondary characters, they are always immigrants in the novel (Puţan 2008, 2010; Marcu 2011). Living in a country, France, that states which is the right path, but itself walks the wrong tracks, the characters, sitting psychologically across a watershed of age (forty years old), understand the West through the rapport of colonizer-colonised, even though they have left the native territory. The new territory is usually Paris, which appears as a very different psychological reality, even unrecognizable, different from the idyllic, touristic image, embellished by the travel agencies, from the vacation adventures or from the melodramatic French and foreign literature of the nineteenth century. The French capital in the novel of the immigrants and expatriates emerges as polymorphous, ethnically coloured, filthy and malodorous, where black, white and Asian people, from the four corners of the Maghreb, search for a better life, a certain welfare for their families. But are they ready to integrate? The relation literature (fiction) and reality (social condition) leans towards a phenomenon well-defined by concepts such as transmigration and bilingualism that the new administrative space, the adoptive country, either assumes or not. From a social point of view, the character and the Romanian narrative landscape mirror the necessity of taking measures and represent a cry of revolt or incapacity/incapability towards some imperious desiderata. Internal state politics and campaigns of awareness raising and information addressed to the general population are promoted more or less intensively. They concern the benefits of foreign citizen integration and the advantages that their participation can bring to the development of the adoptive society, so that the two elements of the equation—immigrant and host—gain from a psychological, identity and economic point of view in the process of individual and statehood becoming. It is not by chance that the target group of such information seminars are members of the local authorities, journalists, opinion leaders, and non-governmental organisations who implement the integration of the immigrants. Culturally, the Romanian character emphasizes the difficulty of the reconciliation between two or more cultures of intersection—here the French culture with that of Maghreb—which consists of the availability of accepting, interiorizing and practicing elements of a culture that the expatriate considers to be foreign, uncomfortable and, above all, betraying the traditions. Here we add the painful phenomenon of bilingualism, so that the identity crisis with its behaviour implications is easy to understand as being part of the direct repercussions of some actions seen as invasive—the child or the youth goes to school with the white people, marries a white person (for instance the Pléthore—Eve Marie marriage in the novel *Beyala*). Between exoticism and curiosity, such literature is the tip of the iceberg of a prestigious social experience in which the francophone writer finds himself in this case, illustrating scripturally by inserting autobiographemes as a sign of his subjectivity. Returning to the immediate reality and eluding the fictional reality, we point out some practical aspects that the literary echoes involve. Demographic European studies monitor the categories of immigrants legally situated on the territory of the member states of the Union, organized or not in the diaspora, and identify the difficulties and the opportunities of the integration process, and announce aspects and models of intervention of the non-governmental organisations regarding the process of social integration. Such measures are wished for and should be amplified, taking into account the fact that the frequent interactions between the immigrants and the autochthonous population have a defining role in the fundamental mechanism of integration, as they prevent negative phenomena such as discrimination, racism or exclusion. Literature, as the mirror of the social phenomenon, refers to the Italian *verismo*, but does not exceed the conceptual boundaries of the movement that Giovanni Verga or Luigi Capuano represent. From the perspective of *verismo*, literature claims its right to represent the whole reality, the way it is, without any idealisation, while the writer no longer invents but records; they are a chronicler, not a creator, and their work competes with the objective reality of the world. Together with Nini's novel, *Ils dissent que je suis une beurette*, and through Samia's character who belongs to the second generation of immigrants, the themes of alienation and loss of identity (Puţan 2011, 60), related to the migration phenomenon, are introduced. Raised between two worlds and two cultures, Samia is a deterritorialized creature, as she knows which one is the origin country of her parents, a place that she has never visited; still, she cannot integrate in the adoptive country since her parents want, at any price and with the risk of alienation, to raise her in the tradition of Maghreb inside the French society, in the Arab diaspora without the girl's consent. In her consciousness, at a stage of moral and axiological development, the Arab-Muslim culture and the culture of the West are not only in religious opposition, but there is also an administrative gap concerning the human rights: if the first is based on millenary traditions and patriarchal primacy, the second invests the woman with the same rights as the man and encourages the feminist movement. This contradiction seen from the point of view of an outsider engenders polemics, controversies or for-and-against dialogues; while seen from the inside it represents a cause of alienation, imbalance, uncertain identities, and psychological deterritorialization. Born in France, Samia bears the stigma of the immigrant—*beurette*—the daughter of immigrants that she cannot understand because she is a French citizen by birth, administratively speaking. She has not yet suffered the rupture from the Arab community for she is forced by her family—meaning the first generation of immigrants—to live by their millenary Muslim rules and customs, carefully preserved in the North African diaspora. Still, Samia is unable to understand the finality, sense and logic of those rules and customs in a society such as France, based on different axiological resources. On the social level, this literary autobiographic exercise casts light on a rapport of reversible vectors. On the one hand, it demonstrates a society that is not prepared to accept and benefit from the presence of foreign citizens, while on the other it incriminates the unprepared immigrants, even those who are part of the second generation, who should integrate in the social time and space that they themselves have chosen. Samia's question "Which one is my country?" triggers the problem of social integration. The interrelated dimensions of this process could be organised in a system of axes, O_{xy} on the vertical, whereas on the horizontal we could have the social and cultural dimensions paired with the economic dimension and public opinion. The first of the four should describe in detail aspects such as the existence of friends, mixed marriages, social, racial, sexual discrimination, stateless people, etc. The second dimension should consider the time spent in the foreign country, the generation born there, the stage of foreign language acquisition (bilingualism would represent a real success of the integration, but not only from an administrative point of view, for, mentally speaking, the writer involves in the fiction and the personal diary usually using his mother tongue), etc. The public opinion dimension should take into account the autochthonous population's view of the foreigners, social representations and expectations, behavioural etiquette and accepted customs, stereotypes, etc. The urban outskirts, as a preferred space of the immigrant, of the stranger, where most of the time they are pushed to and marginalised in the adoptive country, are worth special consideration. In the novel, the territory of the city, negatively marked, and its periphery are places invested with ambiguous connotations; they are open-air prisons, oxymoronically speaking. This type of space is closely related to the psychological identity construction, namely the evolution (or is it the involution?) of the individual, whether they are a fictional character in the novel, or a member of an objective society. Malika and Farida, two female characters in the novel *Beur's Story* by Ferrudja Kessas, live in the outskirts, a place that, in the novel, is regarded as a carceral space (Marcu 2011, 93–98) and a symbol of marginalisation and exclusion of the young immigrants, people also belonging, in this novel, to the second generation. Conceived as a concentric architecture, this place is composed of several circles, differently structured according to their roles in the present and organised according to the scalar principle, going from narrow to vast—the house, the garden, the street, the neighbourhood, the outskirts, the city. If the interior of the house is perceived as a sacred place where the ancestral traditions are kept alive, traditions that have nothing to do with the axiological and moral values of the society in which the family lives (although they should), the street and the neighbourhood which, by superposition, comprise the outskirts, become a space where interpersonal relations seem completely eluded, replaced by misery, unemployment and violence, while the school, the library—situated outside the suburbs—appear as spaces of the breakout from hell. The consciousness of the writer, which can be heard through her characters, operates in the immediate reality with various dichotomies in order to shape this place more accurately: inside/outside, open space/closed space, public space/private space, masculine space/feminine space, real-world space/imaginary space, social space/cultural space. All these types play an essential role in the identity of the characters, who will lay down their lives for their "mistake" of trying to understand why their conservative families do not want or cannot integrate into the French society to which they have emigrated from their origin country. What kind of preparatory activities could the decision factors—first of all the authority of the state—conceive to prevent some negative phenomena such as those described earlier that have premises in the immediate objective reality? Possible, virtual but practical, answers are: an intensive press campaign with communication simulations periodically broadcast in the written local and national press; video clips for television and radio spots; selecting media space providers to broadcast the campaign materials; building teams between partners belonging to different segments of the state: immigration offices, pro-health, pro human rights, pro children's rights foundations and nongovernmental organizations, churches, NGOs, etc. to test the materials created (including the programmes) on the general population. If we were to quantify the relation social phenomenon-literary phenomenon, we can easily realise that the act of reception of a signifying form by the society, be it social or literary, is always a comparative one; that is, we integrate what we have seen and heard into a foregoing, familiar, interconnected and recognisable truth series as we intuitively seek for analogy and the antecedent. That is why we endorse the view that the thing one writes in literature as something plausible goes back to a not-too-distant kind of reality with which the writer starts a dialogue and which the state's authority manages, which sociologists study, psychologists balance out, social workers improve, etc. We deem it necessary to bring to mind the institutional framework of the migration phenomenon whose parameters are in the structure of the EU member states under various forms and names. There should be two axioms on which underpin the social integration implementation: of all the actors involved in the migration phenomenon, the one which defines migration and the legal parameters thereof on its own soil is the state; the management of the migration phenomenon counts on the participation of all the institutions competent for this domain through a participative kind of management and through inter-institutional national and international cooperation, while the leading part falls to the home affairs ministry or the ministry in question; this ministry coordinates a group of institutions which implement the national strategy regarding migration; in turn, these institutions and internal bodies are a part of or are subordinated to certain ministries and governments or are autonomous. Thus, the Ministry of Home Affairs has the following institutions that might launch social programmes for immigrants: the Immigration Office, Border Police Inspectorates, the Foreign Relations Office, the Centre for International Police Cooperation, and the National Agency against Human Trafficking. The Consular Affairs Office is part of the Ministry of Foreign Affairs. On the other hand, the Ministry of Labour might have other institutions accredited to deal with immigrants by taking various steps as those mentioned above: the Labour Employment Department, the National Authority for Child Protection, and the National Authority for Handicapped Persons. A special role falls to the Ministry of Education, which in turn has special departments for pre-university education management as well as for foreign relations and higher education. The General Department for policies, strategies and quality management in health care is a part of the Ministry of Health; in addition to these ministries, the Institute of Statistics, answering directly to the government and the health insurance bodies, serves these persons' interests who, at least temporarily, are members of the social and religious communities and work and live in the adoptive country trying to integrate therein by living up to the values of the state into which they have emigrated.

Conclusions

Janus Bifrons, from the title of our research, refers to the dichotomy immigrant-emigrant as the two faces of the same individual who chooses to live in a geographical and statehood space different from the original space, for a longer or shorter period of time. "Immigrant," is an administrative term related to the country they have chosen to live in, and "emigrant" is a defining element towards one's own consciousness that they are displaced from in an existential familiar location. If literature can be one of the social barometers, then the identity issue, the psychological impasse, the deterritorialisation, the personal crisis, and the (un)assumed bilingualism are aspects that literature brings to the attention of the society through its characters and sees them as emasculating experiences suffered by the immigrant. The competent bodies, the ministries and the national agencies, the institutional media, the social programmes concerning the integration of the immigrants and the checking of the migration flow are instruments of the public authority through which the internal issues, such as those previously described, can be solved, assumed, avoided, and ameliorated in the inward thought process of the immigrant who has the strength to integrate in the community. Starting from a particular case—the francophone novel—we believe that the few considerations made on the literary-social interdisciplinary theme that the sociology of literature mainly deals with are applicable to a larger category of immigrants, not only those coming from Maghreb.

Notes

1 Calixthe Beyala, French writer of Cameroon origin, is the laureate of several important literary prizes: Grand Prix Littéraire de l'Afrique Noire 1993; Prix François Mauriac de l'Académie Française 1994; Grand Prix de l'Académie française 1996; Grand Prix de l'UNICEF 1998.

2 Soraya Nini's novel was published in 1993 in Paris, and filmed in 2000 by the stage director Philippe Faucon, titled *Samia*.

3 The novel of the North African writer of French expression, Ferrudja Kessas, appeared in 1990 through the prestigious printing house L'Harmattan.

References

Marcu, I.-M. (2011). Entre les murs. L'aliénation de l'espace et de l'individu dans le roman *Beur's story* de Ferrudja Kessas [Between the walls: The alienation of the space in the novel *Beur's story*]. *Agapes francophones 2011*. Timişoara: Mirton. 93-110.

Proiectul "Un viitor împreună." Programul general european *Solidaritatea şi gestionarea fluxurilor migratorii.* [The future together. The European programme *Solidarity and management of the migratory flows*]. (2010). Coordinator: Mihai Stoica.

Puţan, I.-M. (2008). L'écriture féminine en Afrique noire: Calixthe Beyala [*Women's writing in black Africa:* Calixthe Beyala]. *Journées de la francophonie 2006-2007*. Timişoara: Mirton. 43-51.

—. (2010). Le sentiment de l'aliénation dans *Ils disent que je suis une beurette* de Soraya Nini [Alienation in Soraya Nini's novel *Ils disent que je suis une beurette*]. In *Agapes francophones* 2010. Timişoara: Mirton. 59-70.

URBAN DEPOPULATION IN ROMANIA: CAUSES AND CONSEQUENCES

DELIA-IOANA NADOLU

Introduction

Social mobility is a very important and consistent process in every society. For the last two decades, Romania's population has continuously decreased for various reasons. This chapter focuses on the demographic evolution of the urban communities of Romania in the last twenty-three years. The population decrease has affected all cities, and there are several main causes for this process: negative natural growth, out-migration, economic changes, urban sprawl, suburbanization, and so on. The consequences are multiple: changes to the work force market, the reconfiguration of urban services, social segregation, housing, brownfields and so on. For this research we used a statistical analysis of the official recorded data from the last two decades concerning the demographical evolution of the entire Romanian urban space (320 cities). As estimated results, the statistical analysis will try to identify some patterns of depopulation and group the cities in several classes related by the causes of depopulation. Starting from these patterns we will describe each cluster and present the main consequences of depopulation.

Theoretical Framework and Methodology

The urban communities represent a contemporary subject, very interesting for various scientific areas, including the urban sociology, social psychology, environmental psychology and cultural anthropology. At the global level, in 2010 the urban population became larger than the rural population (50.9%) (worldbank.org). The high density of urban communities and the accumulation of various kinds of social, economic, technological and cultural resources represent other relevant arguments for the importance of this topic. The city is not just a producer of resources but is also a very consistent consumer of resources. Thus, all over the world any changes in the urban life generate significant consequences for the extended social spaces. When we have to deal with the growing of the city, the entire region follows it on the development trend. On the other hand, when we have to deal with the depopulation of a city the region can also suffer the direct consequences. The shrinking major urban area in North America (Detroit) or the massive shrinking cities of East Germany (Leipzig, Halle, Dresden) represent very eloquent examples of recent urban dynamics that have produced significant effects and were included in the public agenda of local authorities. Following the preliminary results from the last census (2012), the entire Romanian population maintains the trend of the last twenty years in decreasing. From 23,286,794 inhabitants recorded in 1992 the decreasing trend reached the value of 19,042,936 in 2011. Thus, in only two decades the entire population decreased by 18.2% (recensamantromania.ro). Of course, this phenomenon is not unitary at the national level. There are significant differences among the historical regions and between urban and rural communities. Several big cities have reversed the negative trend and started to recover the loss of population, but the differences compared to the 1990s are still significant. From a general point of view, the population decline represents a "normal" stage in the evolution of almost every city. However, the consequences of depopulation are very complex and cannot be ignored, especially by the agenda of local authorities. The manifestations of this phenomenon are connected with the processes of shrinkage, suburbanization and economic revitalization. The depopulation can be correlated with the process of gentrification (Voiculescu 2009; Chelcea 2000). Overall, the presence of these manifestations involves a direct intervention toward urban regeneration. The urban depopulation is a main indicator of the phenomenon of shrinkage. A city affected by shrinkage is not only at risk of depopulation but also from the pressure of other factors. The most important manifestations that can occur with depopulation are:

- Economic and financial problems—the urban depopulation can be directly influenced by the closure of the significant industrial facilities and this usually generates brownfields and an increasing level of unemployment. On the other hand, the urban depopulation generates a decrease in the local budget.
- Problems with urban facilities—the loss of population generates under-use of the entire system of urban facilities (water supply, sewerage), of public transportation, street cleaning, social services, etc.
- House problems—the increase of the vacancy stock, the disequilibria between offer and demand on the estate market, urban sprawl, etc.

- Social problems—the decrease of the population can generate social segregation, gentrification and the alteration of social cohesion.

Considering these aspects our project will focus on the following aspects:

- **Suburbanization** is a very consistent phenomenon directly correlated with the depopulation that has occurred for less than one decade around almost all large cities in Romania. One fully generalized characteristic of this trend is its quasi-chaotic development, without any planned urban scheme. Thus, the cities altered by the artificial communist urbanization process have discovered the possibility of spreading around and toward the closer villages. The urban sprawl assures a relatively quick deintensification of the city centre, but in absence of any architectural master plan the profile of the further suburbs is not based on sustainable principles. In recent years significant "living-room" neighbourhoods were built almost without any urban facilities. Now, the local administrations are trying to recover these gaps and work to extend the public services (as much as possible) and encourage the suburbanization of the commerce and services.
- The **gentrification** process represents another very important topic for various research projects. It can be used as an urban development tool but it directly involves the social segregation process that generates another kind of social problem that also must be solved. In Eastern Europe, after the political changes of 1990, in almost all cities a more or less consistent processes of gentrification occurred, especially against the working class inhabitants with low urban living standards. Even though these examples represent natural reactions of the communist policy to homogenization of the neighbourhoods by mixing populations from various categories, the relocation of the displaced population represents a very important subject with direct consequences for entire communities. Academic discourse has begun to approach the topic (Petrovici 2008) but it is still absent from the public policy.
- **Urban regeneration** represents a somewhat new subject found more frequently in the public discourses of recent years in Romania. The perspectives of developing further metropolitan areas include the urban regeneration of the inner city. Without the upgrading of existing buildings and their urban functionalities, the development of the city is just a theoretical plan. At this level another kind of special problem related to the ownership and use of built spaces is engaged. The public authorities have limited resources to press the private owner to update

their proprieties. The present day legislative system does not allow the city halls to intervene on the real estate market and to apply strategic actions to rebuild the non-functional spaces.

All these main processes, directly correlated with depopulation (urban shrinkage, suburbanization, gentrification, brownfields and urban regeneration), represent relevant contemporary topics for scientific interest and the administrative public policies. The sociological analysis and the main statistical facts can generate a map with patterns of urban depopulation in Romania. The interdisciplinary interpretation of the causes, correlative processes and consequences can offer delimitation between the shrinking cities and sprawling cities. This study is based on a secondary statistical analysis of the official recorded data concerning the evolution of the urban population in Romania.

Results and Discussion

From a general perspective, the Romanian urban population decreased from 1992 to 2012 by 23.3%, from 12,316,439 to 10,054,961. Meantime, the total number of cities increased from 255 to 320 (by transforming 65 large towns into cities). In this twenty-year period Romania lost 4.2 million inhabitants, of which 2.7 million were from urban populations. It is remarkable that most of the cities lost population during this period. The only cities that recorded an increase in population were Buftea (+2,561), Topoloveni (+579), Odovesti (+367), Bolintin Vale (+284) and Mihailesti (+151). In opposition, 50 cities lost more than 30% of their population (from 30% to 50%). We can divide the urban population into three classes: big cities, medium cities and towns (Table 1-1). Following the distribution it is obvious that the medium-sized cities have mostly lost population (26.6%). These cities, with populations between 20,000 and 99,999 inhabitants, are quite different to the rural living style (compared to the towns) and, on other hand, have limited alternatives (for jobs, for living, etc.) compared to big cities. In this category are included the mono-industrial cities (extractive and heavy industries) that where deeply affected by the economic changes of the last two decades. Petrosani had 52,390 inhabitants in 1992 and decreased to 34,331 by 2012 (a decrease of 34.5%), Vulcan from 34,524 to 22,906 (33.7%), and Lupeni from 32,853 to 21,986 (33.1%), etc. From a different perspective, the urban population can be divided by the NUTS II criteria into eight development regions (Table 1-2).

Table 1-1. Classification of the urban population

Type of cities*	Number of cities	Total population	Differences 1992–2012	Difference in %
Big cities (over 100,000 citizens)	24	7,120,715	1,528,801	21.5%
Medium cities (between 20,000 and 99,999 citizens)	82	3,578,769	950,261	26.6%
Towns (below 20,000 citizens)	149	1,616,955	332,741	20.6%

* Counting the volume of population in 1992

Table 1-2. Differences among NUTS II regions

Region	Number of cities*	Total population	Differences 1992 – 2012	Difference in %
1 North-East	31	1,596,462	466,593	29%
2 South-East	33	1,676,226	441,813	26%
3 South	43	1,458,883	331,715	23%
4 South-West	32	1,077,415	238,455	22%
5 West	35	1,302,003	292,787	22%
6 North West	35	1,499,410	270,402	18%
7 Centre	48	1,619,096	383,039	24%
8 Bucharest	3	2,086,944	386,999	19%

* Counting the volume of population in 1992

Table 1-3. Means and standard deviation of depopulation among NUTS II regions

Region	Mean of differences*	Standard Deviation
1 North-East	15,553.10	20,296.009
2 South-East	13,806.66	25,680.649
3 South	7,714.30	10,298.025
4 South-West	7,451.72	11,996.006
5 West	8,365.34	10,209.187
6 North West	7,953.00	10,559.907
7 Centre	7,979.98	14,924.172
8 Bucharest	193,499.50	277,271.418

* Counting the volume of population in 1992

The region with the highest level of depopulation (29%) is the North East, formed by the counties Bacau, Botosani, Iasi, Neamt, Suceava and Vaslui.

From this part of Romania many people have started migrating toward other developed parts of the country or abroad. The region with the smallest level of depopulation (18%) is the North-West with the counties Bihor, Bistrita-Nasaud, Cluj, Maramures, Satu Mare and Salaj (see Table 1-3). Thus, the mean difference between 2012 and 1992 has recorded the lowest level for region 4, with the South-West at 7,451.72. The cities from this region have lost the least population compared to other parts of the country. The highest level of the mean (with the exception of Bucharest) was recorded at 1 by the North East=15,553.10. Thus, in this region, each city was affected by a high level of depopulation.

Conclusions

From 1992 to 2012, the Romanian urban population decreased by 23.3%. Only five cities have recorded a positive trend, and these are the small cities around Bucharest. All other Romanian cities were affected by depopulation. Using different criteria, the higher level of population loss was recorded by the medium-sized cities with a population between 20,000 and 99,000 inhabitants. These cities have a limited number of economic facilities and urban resources and the major changes from the last two decades can produce important effects. From the perspective of NUTS II, the region with the highest level of urban depopulation is the North-Eastern part of Romania. This area has also recorded a high level of out-migration for job opportunities on the European working market.

References

Chelcea, L. (2000). *Grupuri marginale în zone centrale* [Marginal Groups in Central Areas]. *Sociologie Romanească 3-4*: 51-68.

Petrovici, N. (2007). The exclusion of worker families from the city centre of Cluj. Gentrification in a Central-European city. *Romanian Sociology 3*: 13-20.

Voiculescu, S. (Ed.). (2009). *The Romanian Post-socialist City: Urban Renewal and Gentrification.* Timişoara: West University Publishing House

SOCIO-ECONOMIC ASPECTS OF INTERNATIONAL MIGRATION AND DEMOGRAPHIC TRENDS IN ROMANIA

MARIA-ANA GEORGESCU
AND EMILIA HERMAN

Introduction

In the Human Development Reports (HDR) of the United Nations Development Program, according to the composite Human Development Index (HDI), countries are categorized into four groups. A total of 187 countries is divided into three groups of 47 countries with a fourth of 46 at very high HDI, high HDI, medium HDI and low HDI. To assess the level of national development, both economic and social dimensions were taken into account. In the context of HDI rank, the magnitude and complexity of international migration makes it an important force in demographic changes and a high-priority issue for both developing and developed countries.

We noticed in the HD Reports that, with a few exceptions, the net migration rate is positive in the countries characterised as having a very high HDI and has, in general, negative values in the countries with a low HDI. Therefore, the migration fluxes are from the countries in the inferior groups of HDI upward, towards countries with a higher level of HDI.

The present chapter deals with the recent migratory fluxes in the European Union and with the evolution of the international Romanian migration, focusing on the demographic trends.

Our aim is to verify if the factors which determine the general migration flows are validated for the Romanian emigration case and to highlight the implications of massive emigration for the country.

As a **methodology** we used the secondary analysis of many reliable data provided by official international and national statistics and the theoretical approach of the recent migration flows, also regarding the HDI factors which influence this international movement of the population. In this context, we analysed the Romanian emigration fluxes with their destination countries. We realised a comparison between the HDI aspects in these countries and those of Romania. Finally, we put toghether the evolution of Romanian emigration and that of the old age dependency ratio, finding some peculiar aspects regarding the ageing process.

Literature Background

Adopting the decision to migrate, as is well known, has several causes. According to Kandemir (2012, 446), "migrants move to more developed regions in terms of human development." Important emigration fluxes are associated with lower scores of HDI (Sanderson 2009).

Development is a very complex concept. The traditional means of expressing national development have been GDP and level of income. Amatya Sen, winner of the Nobel Prize, in his famous book *Development as Freedom*, believes that development is a process of expanding the real freedoms that people enjoy. The author states that an increase in individual income and GNP is an important way of expanding freedom, but a number of other factors also matter: social issues such as education and social facilities; political issues such as political and civil rights; and technological aspects such as infrastructure modernization. Development requires the removal of major sources that lead to imprisonment, including poverty, tyranny, reduced economic opportunities, neglect of public facilities, intolerance, and repressive governments' excessive control (Sen 2004, 19).

The factor most often cited for migration is revenue size. Given that this fact is related to labour, it would be necessary to "provide some basic training and practical experience for migrant workers in their own countries before they go abroad, because in this way their income potential could double or triple in a short period of time" (Panth 2013).

To synthesize, it is not enough for a country to have a high rate of national income to be considered developed. In this respect, the HDI changed the public and political perceptions of international development (Puentes et al. 2010). According to Kandemir (2012, 446), migrants move to more developed regions in terms of human development, and among the factors which determine migration the most important ones are income, education and health.

European Recent Migratory Fluxes

On the European continent, since 1990 with the fall of the closed totalitarian regimes, a strong population flux from East to West has been registered. This migratory flux aimed at Western Europe is part of a "situation overthrow" that has marked the Old Continent, which once represented the departure point for the highest fluxes of emigrants. It was estimated that during 1850 to 1920, over 50 million Europeans emigrated to America, Australia, India and other areas. Now the western part has transformed into a "terminus point," and Eastern European migration towards Western Europe has acquired a long extension.

The fundamental factors that determine Europe as the continent that absorbed a high number of immigrants are: the decent life conditions, the observance of fundamental freedoms, the huge demand for labour forces, and the perspectives of socio-politic and economic development.

European Union Migration Fluxes

According to official statistics for 2011, there were an estimated 1.7 million immigrants to the EU from a country outside the EU-27 (Eurostat 2013a). Also, 1.3 million people residing inside one of the EU-27 member states migrated to another member state. In total, about 3.2 million immigrants and 2.3 emigrants were reported for the EU-27 Member States.

In 2011, citizens of Romania and Turkey were the most numerous among foreigners in the EU member states, exceeding 2.3 million each.

Comparison between EU Countries Migration Fluxes in 2011

The largest number of immigrants (566,044) were reported by the United Kingdom, and also by Germany (489,422), Spain (457,649) and Italy (385,793); the immigration to these countries represented 60.3% of all inflows to the EU-27 member states (Eurostat 2013a).

More immigration than emigration in 2011 was reported by sixteen of the EU-27 member states, but at the same time in Romania, Bulgaria, the Czech Republic, Ireland, Greece, Spain, Poland and the three Baltic member sates the number of emigrants surpassed the number of immigrants.

For many years, Germany was first regarding the number of immigrants. From 1998, Spain and Italy stood out as having by far the highest net inflows of migrants.

New Citizenship

Migrants, classified according to the level of development of their country of citizenship, based on the HDI, moved from lower ranked countries upward to the countries with higher HDI. As a consequence, a high percentage (52.4%) of all immigrants to the EU were citizens from medium HDI countries, and 34.6% were from high HDI (but non-EU) countries. The migration statistics of Eurostat specify that: "Low HDI countries (6.3 %), EFTA countries (3.6%) and candidate countries (3.1%) accounted for relatively low shares of total immigration to the EU-27 in 2011."

In absolute terms, the main groups of EU citizens acquiring citizenship of another EU member state were: Romanians becoming citizens of Hungary (15,658 persons) and Italy (3,921 persons), Poles becoming citizens of Germany (4,344 persons) and Portuguese becoming citizens of France (3,805 persons).

The largest groups of new citizens in the EU Member States in 2011 were citizens of Morocco (64,200, corresponding to 8.2 % of all citizenships granted) and Turkey (48,800, or 6.2 %).

Evolution of the Romanian International Migration

Situated at fifty-sixth place, Romania is among the countries classified in the second group of HDI. Net Romanian migration rate had a negative value (-0.9). The main destination countries for Romanian outflows can be observed in Table 1-4 below.

Table 1-4. Main destination countries of Romanian emigrants and socio-economic indicators of well-being (2011)

HDI Rank 2011	Destination country	GDP/capita (2005 PPP $)	Public spending (% GDP 2010) Health	Education
Very High HD				
3	USA	42,486	9.5	5.4
5	Germany	34,437	9.0	4.6
11	Canada	35,716	8.0	4.8
23	Spain	27,063	6.9	5.0
25	Italy	27,069	7.4	4.7
High HD				
56	Romania	10,905	4.4	4.3

Our selection from statistical data provided by HDR 2013

According to official country notes, the first ranked countries by the percentage of Romanian emigration fluxes were: Canada (20%), Germany (19%), and the United States (18%), as well as Italy and Spain (Organisation for Economic Co-operation and Development 2013). In these five mentioned countries of destination, the HDI is far higher than in Romania. The reasons why Romanians emigrate are not only economic; they move to countries with better health and education conditions (see Table 1-4).

Non-economic components of human development, like health care quality, education quality and overall life satisfaction, are assessed subjectively. In Table 1-5 below we comparatively observe data collected from 2013 HDR statistics about subjective indicators of well-being.

Table 1-5. Main destination countries of Romanian emigrants and subjective indicators of well-being

HDI rank 2011	**Destination country**	**Satisfaction with health care quality (2007-2009)** % satisfied	**Satisfaction with education quality (2011)** % satisfied	**Overall life satisfaction (2011)** (0 least-10 most satisfied)
Very High HD				
3	USA	56	62.8	7.1
5	Germany	47	65.6	6.7
11	Canada	73	75.4	7.4
23	Spain	84	59.0	6.5
25	Italy	59	46.7	6.1
High HD				
56	Romania	44	45.3	5.0

Our selection from statistical data provided by HDR 2013

Demographic Trends and Implications

In a comparative approach at the European level we notice that the share of old people is bigger than that of youth. The ageing European population is presented here regarding countries.

Official statistics for 2011 reveal that in the EU-27, young people (0 to 14) represented 15.6 % of the population, people considered to be of working age (15 to 64) were 66.9 % of the population, and older persons (65 or over) had a 17.5 % share (Eurostat 2012b).

An illustration of population ageing in EU-27 is provided by the increase of the median age of the population, which increased from 35.2 years in 1990 to 41.2 years in 2011 (Eurostat 2012b).

Population ageing is faster in developing countries than in developed ones (Georgescu & Herman 2010).

As for Romania, our findings highlight a rapid demographic decrease.

Between the two extreme years—1990, with the biggest number of population (23,206,720 inhabitants) and the last available data, and 2011, with the lowest population, (19,043,767 inhabitants)—the difference is about 4,162,953 inhabitants (Table 1-6).

Table 1-6. Evolution of Romanian emigration, of total population and of old age dependency ratio (1990–2011) (thousands of people)

Year	Number of emigrants	Total population	Old age dependency ratio
1990	96,929	23,206.7	15.6
1991	44,160	23,185.1	15.9
1992	31,152	22,810.0	16.6
1993	18,446	22,755.3	16.9
1994	17,146	22,730.6	17.3
1995	25,675	22,681.0	17.6
1996	21,526	22,607.6	18.0
1997	19,945	22,545.9	18.2
1998	17,536	22,502.8	18.7
1999	12,594	22,458.0	19.0
2000	14,753	22,435.2	19.3
2001	9,921	22,408.4	19.6
2002	8,154	21,681.0	20.4
2003	10,673	21,733.6	20.6
2004	13,082	21,673.3	20.9
2005	10,938	21,623.8	21.1
2006	14,197	21,584.4	21.2
2007	8,830	21,537.6	21.3
2008	8,739	21,504.4	21.3
2009	10,211	21,470.0	21.3
2010	7,906	21,431.3	21.4
2011	18,307	19,043.7	21.3

Source: Our selection of data is provided by the Romanian Statistical Yearbook. National Institute of Statistics, 2013 and Eurostat, 2013b

Considering the fact that those who leave are young, in the age group 25–34 *the reproductive capacity decreases*, this being one of the reasons for which the birth rate in Romania is one of the lowest on the continent. The fertility rate in 2011 was 1.25, the lowest in the EU-27 (Eurostat 2012a).

In our country, in comparison to the Western countries which became rich before ageing, the rhythm of demographic ageing has outrun the rhythm of economic development. Moreover, the data available for recent decades have allowed us to foresee the complex economic and social consequences of this ageing on several major directions, such as: economic dependency, impact on the employment of work resources, and impact on economic growth and public expenditure (Georgescu & Herman 2010).

Conclusion

In Romania, one of the developing countries situated in the second category of HDI, the population is decreasing and ageing because of the massive emigration especially of young people and implicitly because of the low fertility rate.

As a demographic trend, the rate of population ageing is higher than the development rate and it matters because the country needs to meet the needs of the older population very fast.

In conclusion, acknowledging these realities only to the extent to which the country will involve the ageing population in the process of goods and services creation (together with other demographic, economic and social policies which are not the subject of this chapter), economic development is possible. Without such a strategy, the macroeconomic disequilibrium will deepen and the demographic ageing will be a permanent obstacle to the growth of the standard of living.

As it concerns the EU-27, economies will surely depend much more on immigration to sustain economic growth. Immigrants are, in general, young people, which is exactly what Europe needs.

References

Georgescu, M.A. & Herman, E. (2010) Aspecte particulare ale îmbătrânirii populaţiei din România post-comunistă—consecinţe socio-economice, [Peculiar aspects of population ageing in the post-communist Romania: Socio-economic consequences]. *Sociologie Românească VIII (4)*: 91-103.

Kandemir, O. (2012) Human Development and International Migration. *Procedia—Social and Behavioral Sciences 62*: 446-451.

Eurostat. (2012a). *Fertility statistics*. Online:

http://epp.eurostat.ec.europa.eu/statistics_explained/index.php/Fertility_statistics.

—. (2012b). *Population structure and ageing*. Online: http://epp.eurostat.ec.europa.eu/statistics_explained/index.php/Population_structure_and_ageing.

—. (2013a). *Migration and migrant population statistics*. Online: http://epp.eurostat.ec.europa.eu/statistics_explained/index.php/Migration_and_migrant_population_statistics.

—. (2013b). *Old age dependency ratio*. Online: http://epp.eurostat.ec.europa.eu/tgm/table.do?tab=table&init=1&plugin=1&language=en&pcode=tsdde510.

National Institute of Statistics. (2013). *Romanian Statistical Yearbook. Time Series 1990-2012*. Online: www.inse.ro.

Organisation for Economic Co-operation and Development. (2013). *Country notes: recent Changes in Migration Movements and Policies*. Online: www.oecd.org/migration/imo.

Panth, B. (2013). Skills Training and Workforce Development with Reference to Underemployment and Migration. In R. Maclean et al. (Eds.), *Skills Development for Inclusive and Sustainable Growth in Developing Asia-Pacific*. Online: http://www.iadb.org/intal/intalcdi/PE/2012/10914.pdf.

Puentes, R., Canales, A., Rodriguez, H., Delgado-Wise, R. & Castles, S. (2010). *Towards an Assessment of Migration, Development and Human Rights Links: Conceptual Framework and New Strategic Indicators*. Online: www.un.org/esa/population/meetings/ninthcoord2011/assessmentofmigration.pdf.

Sanderson, M. (2010). International Migration and Human Development in Destination Countries: A Cross-National Analysis of Less-Developed Countries, 1970-2005. *Social Indicators Research 96 (1)*: 59-83.

Sen, A. (2004). Dezvoltarea ca libertate [Development as Freedom]. Bucureşti: Editura Economică.

United Nations Development Programme. (2013). *Human Development Report: The Rise of South*. Online: http://hdr.undp.org/en/reports/global/hdr2013/.

MODERN FORMS OF SLAVERY: HUMAN TRAFFICKING

FLORENTIN VLAD

Introduction

Human trafficking is a complex phenomenon in today's world, an underground phenomenon of a global dimension that causes millions of human tragedies. However cruel this statement may seem it is real, and human beings are sold and resold at greater and greater costs and exploited like simple objects (Lloyd 2011, 2). Considering the gravity of this phenomenon and the fact that more and more women are becoming the victims of human trafficking after leaving their country with typical dreams for their age, and consequently finding themselves alone among strangers, held prisoner, abused or used as slaves by the traffickers, a warning signal must be provided. Human trafficking, as any other organised crime, is done through a series of crimes. From the moment the victim is recruited, the trafficker and their accomplices break the law multiple times and fundamental human rights are taken away. Most crimes are repeated by the traffickers and are the most serious, damaging the supreme human values of the right to live and freedom. Common assault and bodily injury, homicide, criminal threats and blackmail, forcible confinement and kidnapping, rape and forced prostitution are the offences which are the foundation of trafficking networks. Forgery and fraud, corrupt payments and illegal border crossings are additions to the crimes which the traffickers apply to their destructive plans (Paşca 2011, 99). One must emphasize the fact that victim recruitment in the first stage of trafficking is done through a criminal offence, fraud, in most cases. Although it may seem less grave, the false promise on which a young woman would accept to leave their country is the starting point of all subsequent humiliations and suffering. Human trafficking is one of the gravest offences worldwide because of its social, psychological and moral implications, most of the time having irreparable effects on the whole population—especially children and young people—and also indirectly on the other social categories (Paraschiv 2008, 18). Additionally, it is necessary to find new measures which might reduce these types of crimes.

Methods

The methods used in the drafting of this chapter are analytical and comparative. Statistical data from specialised institutions, NGOs involved in the prevention of human trafficking, and the methods used by criminals were researched through the analytical method. The ways of action of the criminal, the victims' behaviour and the causing factors are researched with the same method. All this is an attempt to analyse different legislative texts with implications in the criminal phenomenon of human trafficking using the comparative method.

Results

Romania is continually making efforts to prevent human trafficking by modifying and adapting the internal legislation so that all of its forms can be punishable, and has founded specialised institutions for prevention, victim protection and repatriation. Since 2001 Romania has adopted a special law for preventing human trafficking which was modified in 2010 to make the fight more efficient (Paraschiv 2008, 22). On the other hand, Romania has reacted rapidly to international measures, always being among the first states to ratify the measures proposed by the European institutions. At present, according to the Romanian Legislation (Law no. 678/2001), the following actions are considered to be human trafficking: the recruitment, transportation, transfer, lodging or accommodation of a person by using threats, violence or other forms of constraint, by kidnapping, fraud, abuse of authority or by taking advantage of another person's inability to protect themself or to express their will, by offering, giving, accepting or receiving money or other goods to obtain the consent of the person with the purpose of exploiting them (Gârbuleț 2010, 67). The analysis of the phenomenon shows that in Romania most victims are from the category of girls and young women aged between 13 and 33 (one quarter of the victims are minors and more than half are aged between 18 and 23). From the young women who were voluntarily repatriated and assisted by the International Organisation for Migration—IOM Office in Bucharest, most of them were taken to Herzegovina, Macedonia, Albania, Kosovo, Italy and Cambodia, and the rest to other countries (Alexandru 2013, 188). Regarding the purpose of human trafficking in certain countries, in Spain, Austria, Germany it is for sexual exploitation, in

Greece for illegal work, and in France and Italy for begging. From the analysis of the way a person becomes the victim of human trafficking, the conclusion is that this process has several stages involving the traffickers, the agents and the victims. The stages of human trafficking are well defined as follows (Gârbuleț 2010, 132):

The recruitment is the moment a "well-wisher," the first element of human trafficking, makes contact with their next victim, making false promises about employment in a foreign country. The victim gives their consent in following the plan of leaving the country of the recruiter. Frequent ways of recruitment are:

- Direct propositions made by acquaintances, relatives, etc.
- Newspaper adverts like: "we recruit young girls, dancers, ballerinas for country X. Immediate departure"; "Professional dances, Cyprus, 2,000 Euros per month, no need for experience, recommendations or dance schools," "Waiters Italy, Spain, Cyprus, Dubai, salaries above 1,500 Euros. We offer lodging for the girls who fought with their parents until the departure," etc.
- False work offers in foreign countries (Italy, Spain, Greece, Austria, Germany) for waiters, chefs on cruise ships, housekeepers or dancers that promise great gains (with some of them masquerading as trips).

What illusions are offered by the recruiters? They promise transportation to the destination, lodging, food, and brag about their "well placed" contacts in other countries.

The **transportation** is organised by the recruiter and is on previously set routes, happening shortly after the recruitment so that the victim doesn't have time to reconsider their decision. The border crossing is often made fraudulently, accompanied by the recruiter and a "guide," and the victim is then delivered to the first buyer, who takes the victim's passport as assurance.

The **sale** is the essence of human trafficking. Victims become merchandise and the buyer-traffickers select them as such. It is only now that the victim is aware of the danger, but the series of sales doesn't usually stop here as the victims are sold successively.

The **exploitation** is total and victims are threatened and abused, subjected to inhuman treatments and sexually exploited as slaves. From the analysis of the victims' declarations who were helped to get back in the country by IOM Bucharest, sustained by a wide sociological study concerning the vulnerability of the female population in Romania towards human trafficking, an outline profile of potential victims has been achieved. In other words, any young woman who sees herself in one of the following situations is more exposed to the dangers of this phenomenon. The big cities in the poor areas of Romania, especially Moldavia (Iaşi, Bacău, Suceava, and Botoşani) and Muntenia, are the main environments for the recruitment of the victims. The victim's origin in a disorganised family or an environment in which the young woman has suffered abuse increases the risk of accepting a false work offer in foreign countries. The low level of education prevents the victim correctly evaluating the information and the plans presented by the recruiter. The triggering factor of the trafficking phenomenon is the decision to leave, along with the unfounded belief that self realization is easier abroad. Such a decision is more likely to appear with persons with difficult financial situations and a lack of opportunities in their own countries (Vechiu 2009, 19). The most vulnerable young women believe that self realization means, first of all, having money, and they are capable of facing danger. The recruitment is done by obtaining the consent of a person in exchange for certain benefits, using situations in which the victim is vulnerable, abuse of power, fraud and sometimes even kidnapping. There are cases when the victims are kidnapped off the street or from different public spaces for entertainment and taken by force into a car. In these extreme cases the recruiters target young women with modest financial situations or someone they know from a disorganised family relying on the fact that no one will be interested in their disappearance (Vechiu 2009, 17). The exploitation includes types of sexual exploitation (Siddharth 2008, 37), work or forced services, slavery or similar practices, and organ harvesting.

Who are the traffickers? They are usually men, but also sometimes women, aged between 20 and 40. Most of them have jobs that lead them to direct contact with victims, such as bartenders, waiters, taxi drivers, etc. They look like trustworthy people and show signs of wealth. They are very convincing and always tell stories about someone who left and accomplished many things abroad. These "well-wishers," willing to help a young woman earn more money, are sometimes acquaintances or even her relatives. When the offer comes from a direct acquaintance, it has to be casual (for example through an encounter at a bar) or vague (from former colleagues or other persons from the past). There are still many citizens, especially young people—who represent the most vulnerable element from the urban and rural environments—who don't truly know the risks that leaving the country presents, something which traffickers count on. The lack of information, as well as a difficult financial situation, is the main factor that encourages trafficking (Bales 2005, 75). Disorganised family origins or an environment where the young woman has suffered abuse increase the risk of accepting a false work offer abroad.

Human trafficking is present worldwide, not only in Romania, and this aspect has resulted from the international institutions' documents (Vechiu 2009, 20). The UNO Office on Drugs and Crime estimates that every minute approximately 2.4 million people are in the process of human trafficking. The International Labour Organisation (ILO) estimates that between the years 2002 and 2011 approximately 20.9 million people were the victims of these networks. The ILO and the European Commission have joined forces to change this phenomenon into a felony for the entire state community.

Discussion

A recent study from the US Embassy in Bucharest showed that the Romanian government has made little effort to protect and assist the victims of human trafficking, despite the fact that the number of identified victims was large.

The government had evidence of 1,041 victims in 2012, and 1,043 victims identified in 2011; 526, approximately half of the total number of victims, were trafficked for sexual exploitation, while 410 were trafficked for forced work. Other victims were forced to beg, steal and participate in the making of pornographic material. The number of victims who were children went up from 319 to 370 in 2012; 492 of the victims were trafficked in the country's territory.

The main problems in fighting human trafficking are legislative deficiencies, the lack of education and information, and the lack of efficient institutions which would identify these crimes.

The European Parliament and Council have enacted the Directive 2011/36 concerning human trafficking and the victims' protection from it since April 5, 2011, and the member states were obliged to implement it until April 6, 2013, and then in 2016 to make an evaluation of its impact. In April 2013, Cecilia Malmström, the European Commissary of Internal Affairs, announced that only 9 of the 27 states have implemented these stipulations in the national legislation—the Czech Republic, Poland, Latvia, Lithuania, Estonia, Finland, Hungary, Sweden and Romania—and 4 other states have implemented them partially—Belgium, Bulgaria, Slovenia and the United Kingdom. The implementation of the directive is essential to have a common legal framework to define the crime of trafficking in persons, to punish those found guilty and guarantee protection of the witnesses.

Romania's efforts are not final. Thus, the Ministry of Administration and the Interior has announced the creation of The Integrated System of Monitoring and Evaluation of the Human Trafficking Victims (SIMEV), and the issue of human trafficking has been included in the Government Program 2012 in the 2nd addendum of the Parliament's decision no. 15/2012 for trusting the Government, in chapter 6 "Administration and the Interior," where criminality, human trafficking, drug trafficking and contraband are presented as the only dangers of the interior safety of Romania, against which the public institutions in the field of order and safety must take adamant measures co-ordinately with other European authorities.

The Romanian Government has improved the efforts in preventing human trafficking by continuing the development of intense campaigns of raising awareness and by coordinating a national strategy and a plan of action for fighting human trafficking. The National Agency against Trafficking in Persons continued to develop policies referring to human trafficking and the national mechanism in reference to institutions. With this purpose, the agency has collaborated with NGOs to elaborate a national strategy to fight against human trafficking between 2012 and 2016 and a plan of action between 2012 and 2014. In 2012, the government has launched six national and regional campaigns and thirty-six local campaigns to inform people in secondary and high schools, putting billboards in bus stations, on screens in subway stations, at cinemas and on the internet. A modification of the Criminal Code in 2006 forbids the recruiter companies registered in Romania to enable the exploitation of citizens in foreign countries, but the authorities haven't penalised any company for human trafficking activities so far.

What should be done for an efficient fight against human trafficking? First of all, they should offer more finance for the assistance of programs for human trafficking victims, including funding NGOs which offer different services to the victims (Alexandru 2013, 288).

Another option would be raising the quality of services offered to victims, ensuring a considerable attendance through psychological guidance, rehabilitation and other assistance activities offered to the victims.

Last but not least, they should build shelters exclusively for the victims of human trafficking who were repatriated and eliminate the restrictions of movement imposed on the victims during their placement in the government financed centres, supposing this doesn't affect the victims' safety.

The improvement of the efforts of identifying the potential victims among the vulnerable categories of the population, like immigrants without identification documents, foreign workers, the Roma population and the children who beg or practice prostitution, is another objective which should be achieved.

Acknowledgement

This work was partially supported by the strategic grant POSDRU/ CPP107/DMI1.5/S/78421, Project ID 78421 (2010), co-financed by the European Social Fund—Investing in People, within the Sectoral Operational Programme Human Resources Development 2007–2013.

References

Alexandru, M. L. (2013). *Asistența și reintegrarea socială a victimelor traficului de persoane* [Assistance and Social Integration of Human Trafficking Victims]. București: Editura Universității din București.

Bales, K. (2005). *Understanding Global Slavery: A Reader*. Berkeley, CA: University of California Press.

Council Directive 2004/81/EC of 29 April 2004 on the residence permit issued to third-country nationals who are victims of trafficking in human beings or who have been the subject of an action to facilitate illegal immigration, who cooperate with the competent authorities. *Official Journal L 261, 06/08/2004 P. 0019—0023.*

Council of Europe. (1983). *European Convention on the Compensation of victims of violent crimes*. Strasbourg.

Decision No 779/2007/EC of the European Parliament and of the Council of 20 June 2007 establishing for the period 2007-2013 a specific programme to prevent and combat violence against children, young people and women and to protect victims and groups at risk (Daphne III programme) as part of the General Programme Fundamental Rights and Justice. *Official Journal L 173, 3.7.2007:* 19-26.

Directive 2011/36/EU of the European Parliament and of the Council of 5 April 2011 on preventing and combating trafficking in human beings and protecting its victims, and replacing Council Framework Decision 2002/629/JHA. *Official Journal L 101/1, 15.04.2011.*

Gârbuleț, I. (2010). *Traficul de persoane* [Human Trafficking].București: Universul Juridic.

Legea nr. 211 din 27 mai 2004 privind unele măsuri pentru asigurarea protecţiei victimelor infracţiunilor. *Monitorul Oficial, Partea I nr. 505 din 4 iunie 2004.*

Legea nr. 286 din 17 iulie 2009—Codul Penal. *Monitorul Oficial, Partea I nr. 510 din 24 iulie 2009.*

Legea nr. 678 *din 21 noiembrie 2001* privind prevenirea şi combaterea traficului de persoane. *Monitorul Oficial, Partea I nr. 783 din 11 decembrie 2001.*

Lloyd, R. (2011). *Girls Like Us: Fighting for a World Where Girls Are Not for Sale*. London: Harper Collins Publishers.

Paraschiv, G. (2008). *Traficul de persoane* [Human Trafficking]. Bucureşti: Ars Academica.

Paşca, V. (2011). *Studii de drept penal* [Criminal Law Studies]. Bucureşti: Universul Juridic.

Recommendation R(85)11 of the Committee of Ministers to Member States on the position of the victim in the framework of criminal law and procedure, adopted by the Committee of Ministers on the 28th June 1985 at the 387th meeting of the Ministers' Deputies.

Siddharth, K. (2008). *Sex Trafficking: Inside the Business of Modern Slavery.* New York, NY: Columbia University Press.

Vechiu, A. (2009). *Traficul de persoane* [Human Trafficking]. Iași: Lumen.

Human Trafficking and the Infringement of European Values

Beniamin Lup

Introduction

Human trafficking has become the phenomenon of the century by destroying individuals, families and communities. We should look at human trafficking and its consequences on its victims, their families and nations, and we should evaluate and see how this, once referred to in a title of a book as "a crime so monstrous," became the slavery of the modern age. In this chapter we will see how our efforts to build a United Europe are infringed by organized crime. We will see how the values on which Europe was founded, and the principles the European Union was built, are attacked by this shameful phenomenon which tries to grow under our very eyes. It denies people their human rights and dignity, freedom of choice and movement and protection of life; it refuses to ensure equality among people and quality of life. As we consider these, we are challenged to act now. Through the laws we elaborate and pass, we are all responsible for combatting this monstrous crime. Through our influence we are called on to inform the world about the danger of this phenomenon, and through the actions we take to pursue the goals which the founders of the European Union once had: freedom for all, equality of all, dignity and responsibility.

Jacques Delors was the president of the European Commission. Just before his term of office expired, in 1992, he wrote a letter to the religious leaders across Europe pleading for them to help recover the soul of Europe, and to help shape its future. Was the soul of Europe saved? Are we still waiting for a response? Have you answered the call? Delors wrote:

> If in the ten years ahead of us we do not succeed in giving Europe its soul, a spiritual dimension, true significance, then we will have been wasting our time. That is the lesson of my experience. Europe cannot live by legal argument and economic know how alone. The potential of the Maastricht

> Treaty will not be realized without some form of inspiration. (Summary of Addresses by President Delors to the Churches)

The founding fathers of the European Union were certainly inspired by ideals, objectives and values that transcended and animated legal and economic integration. One of them, Robert Schuman, put it this way in 1950:

> We are called to bethink ourselves of the Christian basics of Europe by forming a democratic model of governance which through reconciliation develops into a "community of peoples" in freedom, equality, solidarity and peace and which is deeply rooted in Christian basic values. (Déclaration du 9 mai 1950)

The European Union was created as a supranational foundation to make war unthinkable and materially impossible, and to reinforce democracy. The Europe Declaration was a joint statement issued by the Foreign Ministers of Germany, France, Italy, the Netherlands, Belgium and Luxembourg, and it said that the community marked the birth of Europe as a political, economic and social entity, reflecting the principles that Schuman announced in the Schuman Declaration, including the statement:

> By the signature of this Treaty, the participating Parties give proof of their determination to create the first supranational institution and that thus they are laying the true foundation of an organised Europe. This Europe remains open to all European countries that have freedom of choice. We profoundly hope that other countries will join us in our common endeavour. (Sahm 1951)

The founders of the European Union believed in the Values of respect for human dignity, liberty, democracy, equality, the rule of law, and for human rights (Article I-2, The European Declaration)

As the union grew and member states were added to the European family its "enemies" became active. Besides the economic and political challenges, social phenomena became a reason for concern. Organized crime and networks of criminal structures were threatening the great plans for a common and united entity, and corruption and greed caused many people to harm others. The differences between the judicial systems became reasons for some to be concerned, and for others became ways to take advantage of people. Albert Einstein once said: "It has become appallingly obvious that our technology has exceeded our humanity." The fast development of technology was used by criminal organizations infringing every concept of humanity and freedom. Surveys tell us that organized crime increases around the world like a plague. The Global Report on Trafficking in Persons launched by the United Nations Office on Drugs and Crime (UNODC) provides new information on a crime that shames us all. According to this report, the most common form of human trafficking (79%) is sexual exploitation. The victims of sexual exploitation are predominantly women and girls. Worldwide, almost 20% of all trafficking victims are children. The EU Strategy towards the Eradication of Trafficking in Human Beings 2012–2016 contains this report:

> Trafficking in human beings takes many different forms, and evolves with changing socioeconomic circumstances. It targets women and men, girls and boys in vulnerable positions. The latest estimates from the International Labour Organization of June 2012 covering the period 2002–2011 put the number of victims of forced labour, including forced sexual exploitation, to 20.9 million at a global level, with an estimated 5.5 million children being trafficked. However, this estimate is also believed to be conservative. A lucrative form of crime, trafficking in human beings generates profits of dozens of billions of euro for the perpetrators each year. (Belser 2005)

> Most people think that slavery is a crime of the past. However, this notion couldn't be any further from the tragic reality of a well organized criminal activity which victimized more than 30 million women and children worldwide. As matter of fact, there are more people being enslaved today than at any other time in human history. There are two distinct facets of this modern slave trade: one concerns victims who are sold, bought and used as sex slaves, the other one pertains to people exploited for labour purposes … Sophisticated criminal organizations are exploiting a situation of despair created by a global system where human beings are not much more than a resource and a commodity. (Mercier 2012)

Different sources have presented definitions of human trafficking, being described from legal, sociologic, religious, economic and political perspectives, and different organizations have come up with different definitions. The truth is that:

> … there is no universally accepted definition of trafficking for sexual exploitation. The term encompasses the organized movement of people, usually women, between countries and within countries for sex work with the use of physical coercion, deception and bondage through forced debt. However, the issue becomes contentious when the element of coercion is removed from the definition to incorporate facilitating the willing involvement in prostitution. (en.wikipedia.org/wiki/Human_trafficking)

Article 3, paragraph (a) of the **Protocol to Prevent, Suppress and Punish Trafficking in Persons** defines Trafficking in Persons as the recruitment, transportation, transfer, harbouring or receipt of persons, by means of the threat or use of force or other forms of coercion, of abduction, of fraud, of deception, of the abuse of power or of a position of vulnerability or of the giving or receiving of payments or benefits to achieve the consent of a person having control over another person, for the purpose of exploitation. The **United Nations** defines human trafficking as:

> … the recruitment, transportation, transfer, harbouring or receipt of persons, by means of the threat or use of force or other forms of coercion, of abduction, of fraud, of deception, of the abuse of power or of a position of vulnerability or of the giving or receiving of payments or benefits to achieve the consent of a person having control over another person, for the purpose of exploitation.

The "slavery market" adds two million new victims of human trafficking every year. This twenty-first century slavery ruins individual lives, families and nations. Europe is facing a growing movement of organized crime related to human trafficking. State members write policies and spend a considerable amount of funds preventing the crime and prosecuting the criminals. Many NGOs spend thousands of hours in voluntary work to counsel the victims and rehabilitating them for reinsertion into the society. National institutions spend great funds on providing for victims and their families. Sometimes, it seems that things are out of control. The European Union has developed mechanisms for the legislation of the member states to prevent, slow and/or combat the criminal activity in this area. Conferences, resolutions, seminars and campaigns are all designated to stop the growth of this modern slavery. International bodies have addressed trafficking and counter-trafficking measures in a variety of declarations, resolutions and other instruments, such as:

- The Universal Declaration of Human Rights 1948
- The Declaration on the Rights of the Child 1959
- The Vienna Declaration and Programme of Action of the World Conference on Human Rights 1993
- The Declaration on the Elimination of Violence against Women 1993
- Programme of Action of the International Conference on Population and Development, Cairo 1994
- World Summit for Social Development, Copenhagen 1995.

The United National General Assembly has, since 1993, adopted a series of resolutions on Trafficking in Women and Girls and on the Need to Adopt Efficient International Measures for the Prevention and Eradication of the Sale of Children, Child Prostitution and Child Pornography, and on Measures for the Prevention of Smuggling of Aliens. The Economic and Social Council has adopted a series of resolutions, such as the Resolution on Measures to Prevent Illicit International Trafficking in Children and to Establish Penalties Appropriate to Such Offenses (1996), the Resolution on Action against Illegal Trafficking in Migrants, Including by Sea (1998), the Resolution on Action to Combat International Trafficking in Women and Children (1998), and the Resolution on the Human Rights of Migrants (1999). The commission of Human Rights adopted in 1996 several resolutions on "Traffic in Women and Girls," "Contemporary Forms of Slavery" and the "Rights of the Child," whereby governments, intergovernmental and nongovernmental organizations and other bodies are called on to continue and develop new measures to combat trafficking in women and children. From the office of the Secretary General and the office of the High Commissioner of Human Rights, several reports on Trafficking in Women and Girls have been released. INTERPOL adopted in 1996 a resolution on "Traffic in Human Beings and the International Exploitation of Prostitution," recommending a multidisciplinary, cooperative approach regarding the sharing of information and other activities aimed at combatting trafficking, exploitation of prostitution and illegal marriages.

Steve Harvey, the Acting Head of Europol's Operations Department Unit, states that the scale of organized crime in the EU is considerable and that trafficking in human beings is one of the most prevalent organized crime activities. The EU offers an attractive consumer base for organized crime, with half a billion relatively affluent citizens, liberalized markets, an enterprising business culture and freedom of movement facilitated by the Schengen Agreement. Steve Harvey underlines that "an effective EU response should address the problem in a holistic way," recognizing its transnational features and its growing complexity:

> A common integrated architecture is required, promoting joint operations between the member states and EU agencies against the highest priority threats, including trafficking in human beings. Tackling human trafficking should not be seen solely as a domestic challenge for the member states. The investigation of human trafficking needs to recognize the almost ever present international elements, and investigations should be seen as integral to the international efforts to combat trafficking specifically and organized crime in general. (Harvey 2010)

We will discuss some of the values the European Union is built upon, and see how these values are infringed in general by organized crime and in particular by trafficking in persons. The official reports are just glimpses of what the reality of this phenomenon is. In 2002, the International Organization for Migration estimated that as many as 20,000 women were trafficked from Romania each year; according to some estimates, 10–15% were minors (Hamburg Institute of International Economics 2007). Between 2005–2007, the rate of female victims being trafficked to Western Europe for sexual exploitation was the highest in Romania of all countries in Eastern Europe. In 2008, Romanians were identified as victims of trafficking in twenty-three countries around the world. In 2009, The U.S. State Department reported in its Trafficking in Persons Report that:

> Romania is a source, transit, and destination country for men, women, and children subjected to forced labour and women and children subjected to sex trafficking. Romanian men, women, and children are subjected to forced labour in agriculture and manufacturing, as well as some forced inot begging in Spain, Italy, the Czech Republic, Greece, Finland, Israel, Germany, Slovenia, the United Kingdom, Cyprus, Australia, France, Belgium, and the United States. A large proportion of the children of Roma ethnicity are forced to beg in Western European countries. Men, women, and children from Romania are victims of forced prostitution in Italy, Sweden, Spain, the Netherlands, the United Kingdom, Greece, Germany, Cyprus, Austria, Switzerland, Czech Republic, Denmark, Brazil, Norway, Hungary, Slovenia, and France. Forced labour and sex trafficking within the country claim Romanian men, women, and children as victims; this includes forced begging and forced petty theft. (U.S. State Department 2009)

Although the US Department of State commended Romania for its progress in preventing and combatting human trafficking, in the 2012 report on human trafficking it had some recommendations:

- Restore government funding for trafficking victim assistance programs, including grants for NGOs providing service to victims
- improve the quality of victim services, ensuring that psychological care, rehabilitation and other victim assistance provide substantive care
- construct a trafficking specific shelter for repatriated victims in Bucharest
- remove non-security related restrictions on victims' movement while housed in government-funded shelters

- encourage male trafficking victims to use assistance to prevent further exploitation
- adopt stronger measures for the long-term rehabilitation of child victims who are vulnerable to re-trafficking
- ensure that reintegration and rehabilitation of child victims address any parental involvement in the original trafficking of the child
- improve the reporting of data on trafficking crimes prosecuted under Law No. 678/2001 and other relevant laws by disaggregating sex and labour trafficking offenses; explore ways to improve asset confiscation and victim compensation; vigorously investigate and prosecute acts of trafficking-related complicity allegedly committed by government officials, and punish officials convicted of such crimes with prison sentences
- consider specialized training for labour inspectors in identifying trafficking cases; demonstrate efforts to investigate and punish acts of labour trafficking and efforts to assist victims of labour trafficking
- ensure protection of trafficking victims during trial by making sustainable plans and funding for victims' appearances in pre-trial hearings and travel to trial
- reduce delays in trials
- improve efforts to identify potential victims among vulnerable populations, such as undocumented migrants, foreign workers, Roma, and children involved in begging or prostitution
- consider offering foreign trafficking victims the right to work during the duration of their temporary residence permits
- continue to provide victim sensitivity training for judges (state.gov).

Human trafficking becomes a more and more obvious threat to the world. Every value of the European Union is clearly meant for the benefit of every person, and member states are making efforts to ensure the social peace for the citizens of the EU. On the other hand, organized crime and trafficking infringe on every value.

Human rights and human dignity

Deeply rooted in the Bible and the Christian Tradition, the concept of human dignity triggers the concept of human rights. There can be no human rights without the belief that human beings are created with dignity. Human dignity originates from God and is of God because we are made in God's own image and likeness. Genesis 1: 26–27 teaches that human life is sacred because the human person is the most central and clearest reflection of God among us. Human beings have transcendent worth and value that comes from God; this dignity is not based on any human quality, legal mandate or individual merit or accomplishment. Human dignity is inalienable, meaning thatit is an essential part of every human being and is an intrinsic quality that can never be separated from other essential aspects of the human person.

Freedom of choice

The international treaties are means through which individuals are guaranteed to be free to make their own choices. The inner value of each person entitles individuals to be able to choose and bear the consequences of their choices. Freedom to choose makes humans special and different in the animal world. Human trafficking infringes the right of persons to act based upon their own choice. Furthermore, victims are often punished to bear the consequences of someone else's choice (the criminal), sometimes for a lifetime. There is no freedom of choice for the mother promised a good job who is taken away from her children and forced into slavery. There is no freedom of choice for the young girl abducted by a criminal or a criminal network and forced into sexual bondage. There is no freedom of choice for the little kids forced to become beggars and work long hours in misery and harsh conditions. There is no freedom of choice for the human used for organ harvesting.

Freedom of Movement

Every day, scores of young women throughout the former Soviet Bloc are lured by job offers that lead to a hellish journey of sexual slavery and violence. Despite the barrage of warnings on radio and TV, in newspapers and on billboards, desperate women continue to line up with their naiveté and applications in hand, hoping that this time they might just be in luck. Once a person becomes a victim of human trafficking, his or her freedom of movement is infringed. Our organization, WorldTeach, works hard with victims of human trafficking. The abuses, beatings and limitations forced upon them while they were trafficked has impacted their behaviour hugely. They are afraid to travel, afraid to make choices and afraid to take initiative even months or years after being released from captivity and harassment.

Protection of life

Life is the most precious gift given unto us as human beings. The oldest laws of humankind protected life. The law of Moses, given thousands of years ago, clearly protected life in all stages until natural death. The Bible clearly speaks against murder, exploitation and commerce with human beings. Human trafficking infringes the right to life and the protection that laws guarantee. Children and adults alike are robbed of their elementary right to a decent life. All victims are abused and often lose their lives. Their health and life are endangered, and quality of life is always threatened by human trafficking. Destroying individuals, families, communities and nations, trafficking destroys life and its essence. As a gift from God, every human life is sacred from conception to natural death. The life and dignity of every person must be respected and protected at every stage and in every condition. The right to life is the first and most fundamental principle of human rights that leads us to actively work for a world of greater respect for human life and greater commitment to justice and peace (usccb.org).

Equality

Nobody should consider himself of herself above other people in order to take advantage of them. Adults and children, men and women, are all equal in nature, value and dignity. They are equally entitled to spiritual and physical development. No one can oppress others under any circumstances. No one is above others as we were created by the same creator and given the same spirit of life. Human trafficking steals people's deepest desire and hinders their strongest dreams of succeeding in life.

Conclusion

The United Nation's International Labour Organization's 2012 Estimate on Forced Labour provides some shocking statistics on the prevalence of human trafficking worldwide:

- Of the 20.9 million victims of trafficking and human slavery worldwide, 9.1 million victims (44%) have been trafficked internally or internationally.
- 11.8 million are subjected to forms of modern slavery in their place of origin or residence within their own national borders.

- Nearly 1.5 million victims are currently labouring in conditions of forced labour, sexual exploitation and servitude in the United States, Canada and developed countries of the EU.
- .55 percent of forced labour victims are women and girls, as are 98 percent of sex trafficking victims.
- Children aged 17 years and below represent 26 percent of total victims, representing a total of 5.5 million child victims worldwide.

This could lead us to state that Human Trafficking is the most horrible crime the world has known. It infringes every principle and every value of any society and culture. It destroys lives of individuals, families and nations. As a threat to global, national and individual security, trafficking in persons must be tackled collectively through a human security approach that advocates for comprehensive, people-centred, context-specific and preventive solutions. Placing people, and the conditions in which they live, at the centre of analysis, the human security concept argues for not only the physical safety of the affected individuals, groups and communities but also addresses the root causes behind human trafficking. (Lup, 2011) For example, by considering the relevant threats to the survival, livelihood and dignity of the affected individuals and communities, the human security concept can highlight the underlying cultural, social, political and economic root causes behind human trafficking and advance the necessary partnerships required to tackle this multifaceted global threat. As we consider these, we cannot stand the challenge to act now. Through the laws we elaborate and pass, we are all responsible to combat this monstrous crime. Through our influence we are called to inform the world about the danger of this phenomenon. Through the actions we take we are called to pursue the goals which the founders of the European Union once had: freedom for all, equality of all, dignity and responsibility. The attitude of William Wilberforce could be a challenge for us all. He once said:

> "If to be feelingly alive to the sufferings of my fellow-creatures is to be a fanatic, I am one of the most incurable fanatics ever permitted to be at large. You may choose to look the other way but you can never again say you did not know." (*William Wilberforce's 1789 Abolition Speech*)

Schuman stated in his Declaration of May 9, 1950:

> "World peace cannot be safeguarded without the making of creative efforts proportionate to the dangers which threaten it." (http://www.robert-schuman.eu/declaration_9mai)

We are called to restore the soul of Europe and the values its founders stood for. We are called to act before too late.

Acknowledgement

This work was possible with the support of WorldTeach Team and the Bridge to Europe Foundation. Their contribution to the prevention of human trafficking and their investments into the lives of victims and their families make a great difference in this world.

References

Belser, P. (2005). *Forced Labour and Human Trafficking: Estimating the Profits.* Geneva: International Labour Office.

Commission of the European Communities. (1992). *Summary of Addresses by President Delors to the Churches*, Nr. 704E/92.

Cornilescu, D. (Ed.). (1923). *Biblia* [The Bible]. Bucureşti.

European Commission. (2012). *The EU Strategy towards the Eradication of Trafficking in Human Beings 2012-2016*. Brussels.

gotQuestions?org. Online: http://www.gotquestions.org/human-trafficking.html.

Harvey, S. (2010). Monitoring mechanisms in the fight against human trafficking. Online: http://www.nyc.gov/html/endht/downloads/pdf/monitoring_mechanisms_final_report.pdf.

Human Trafficking. Online: http://en.wikipedia.org/wiki/Human_trafficking.

ILO Global Estimate of Forced Labour 2012: Results and Methodology. Online: http://www.ilo.org/washington/WCMS_182004/lang--en/index.htm

Lup, B. (2012). *WorldTeach, ONGurile si prevenirea traficului de fiinte umane. Perspective multidisciplinare asupra prevenirii si combaterii traficului de persoane* [WorldTeach, NGOs and the Prevention of Human Trafficking: Multidisciplinary Perspectives on the Prevention and Control of Human Trafficking]. Cluj-Napoca: Cordial Lex.

Mercier, G. (2012). Human Trafficking: Modern Day Slavery. *News Junkie Post*, 15 Feb 2012.

Sahm, Ul. (1951). *Der Schuman Plan. Vertrag ueber die Gruendung der europaeischen Gemeinschaft fuer Kohl und Stahl* [The Schuman plan. Agreement on the creation of the European Coal and Steel Community]. Frankfurt.

Schuman, R. (1950). *Déclaration du 9 mai*. Online: http://www.robert-schuman.eu/declaration_9mai.

Skinner, B. (2009). *A crime so monstrous*. New York, NY: Free Press.

U.S. Department of State. Diplomacy in Action. Online: http://www.state.gov/documents/organization/192597.

U.S. State Department. (2009). *Trafficking in Persons Report,* June 2009.

William Wilberforce's 1789 Abolition Speech. Online: http://www.brycchancarey.com/abolition/wilberforce2.htm.

CHAPTER TWO

CONSTRUCTION OF IDENTITY

MIGRATION AND SOCIAL INTEGRATION: THE ROMA IN THE EU

CLAUDIA-ANAMARIA IOV

"The Roma issue" appeared on the international arena as a threat to the European geopolitical stability due to the successive migration waves, of the economic, political and social effects driven by repatriation agreements and financial support for them, professional and social reinsertion programs, and international treaties for human and minority rights, and especially the great number of actors involved in addressing this situation, such as the origin state, reception states, international profile organizations and Roma community leaders.

The question we start from is related to the impact of the enlargement process and the immigration on the EU policies. To what extent do the eastern immigrants (especially economic immigration) effect the relations between immigrants—states—and international actors? What is the effect of the Roma migration case on the debate enlargement vs. European political integration? The issue has two dimensions: the current situation, for which resolution policies and programs are formulated; and the potential problem due to an increased visibility of the enhanced Roma migration from the eastern and south-eastern European countries (especially Romania, Bulgaria, Slovakia or the states in Western Balkans) towards the developed countries of Western Europe, which unfortunately are still facing the prolonged effects of the economic crisis and its social and political consequences.

A recent topic—especially after the last extension wave of the EU encompassing Romania and Bulgaria, countries with a significant number of Roma—is fear of the "gypsy invasion" from the East in the developed states of the EU as part of a greater issue, namely "the fear of immigrants," a widespread phenomenon within but not limited to Western Europe. This problem worsened due to the economic crisis, and the most vulnerable of the immigrants became scapegoats, because those states did not manage the economic crisis effects correctly or they were used as an election campaign theme, being closely connected to the national security issue (see the case of France in the 2012 elections). From our point of view, it is difficult to draw final conclusions at this moment, mostly because a project of "zero migration for Roma" is impossible, and on the other hand a coherent Roma social integration project is not yet available on the "EU market."

In this analysis, migration must be understood and regarded as a spill-over effect, bringing together previous sectors of analysis that were studied separately. In the current context, marked by economic crisis, migration has been elevated to the level of meta-issue (Bigo 2001, 121–122), and the boundaries between threats to internal and external politics become more ambiguous.

The analysis refers to the migration-identity-security relationship, but does not require an exhaustive analysis of the migration phenomenon in the EU (which includes both the immigrants in the member states and those in the third-party states). Our analysis framework will only be applied to the migration between the EU member states with a focus on "the existential threats" from the Roma, who bring forward a xenophobic and racist past of the twentieth century Europe (see the situation of the Roma during the Holocaust) within a larger debate on expansion vs. European integration.

Since 2001 (after the beginning of "the war against terrorism") we can observe an increase in representation incidence and association of immigrants and asylum seekers with issues related to terrorism, organized crime, threats to national identity or sovereignty. Their visibility is determined by the great number of incidents in the majority population or by the host state's inability to integrate them. An important role is also played by the subjective nature of the construction of the two concepts of security and migration, taking into account the interest of the actor who securitizes: "migration, security and the linkage between the two of them [being] inherently subjective concepts [which depend on the interest of the one who] is defining the terms and who benefits by defining the terms in a given way" (Choucri 2002, 98).

In the context of globalization, the relationship migration-security takes on new dimensions with ample reverberations in the economic, political, social, demographic and societal fields. Globalization draws a new era rising from the ruins of the Cold War period, feeding on a worldwide economy turning global under the pressure of massive technology, telecommunication and cross-continental transport development.

Migration is not a new phenomenon, emerging with the states and simultaneously developing with them. Nowadays, the East-West, South-North migration has intensified and diversified against the economic development and necessity for a cheap labour force, as presented in the charts below. The EU expansion (especially the waves of 2004 and 2007) has led to "the increase of migratory influxes from east to west, especially from Central and Eastern Europe, but also Central Asia and Africa, towards the West" (Sarcinschi 2008, 5). The frequency of immigrant waves in the EU states depends on a series of factors, among which are the accession of new members (determining an explosion in the number of immigrants willing to take advantage of the benefits offered by EU member state status), a seasonal labour demand (in the summer and autumn there is an increased number of economic immigrants), and the effects of economic recession (the economic crisis determined a part of the economic immigrants to return to their states of origin/or change the destination state in search of another work place).

The east-west migration and the ethnic minorities' movement became greater and highly mediatised due to unfortunate events between the immigrant and the majority populations within destination countries (for example, the Mailat case in Italy, the situation of the Roma in France 2010–2012, Northern Ireland 2009, the Hungarians in southern Austria, the Turks in Germany, etc.). Policymakers have used these incidents in their struggle for power and financial resources, turning the migration (legal and illegal), refugees and asylum seekers' issues into a meta-issue, a game of power with comprehensive economic, social and societal reverberations.

There are several levels of analysis on the migration-security relationship, but of these the two we present in our analysis present migration, in the first instance, as a result of insecurity (mainly military, but also economic), while the second level presents migration as a source of insecurity (political, economic, military or societal) (Ibid., 11). The effects of this relationship, regardless of the level of analysis, are perceived (on political, economic, social and societal levels) by all the actors involved, namely the immigrants, the majority population, the state of origin, the destination state, the media, the profile of international organizations and interested social actors.

Migration itself is not an insecurity phenomenon; however, uncontrolled and illegal migration has destabilizing effects on the international security system. In the face of such danger, being unable to unilaterally stop the migratory influx, the state delegates certain political powers towards the supranational level, particularly towards the European Commission and the European Parliament. As we have also observed in the case of the Roma in France, the French state assumed the role of securitization actor, and the EU, through its institutions, of desecuritization actor. The confrontation, based on the legitimacy of the intervention, takes place between the French national interest and the basic principles of European integration, which have always aimed at ensuring a secure environment in Europe.

Migration as a result of insecurity is a phenomenon that mainly occurs at moments of tension, following military conflicts that involve waves of refugees to neighbouring or triumphant states (the First and Second World Wars, the Holocaust, the war in the Western Balkans states, the Arab Spring, etc.), or with political regime changes, such as the fall of communism or the "Arab Spring," which led to an increase in migration towards the developed and economically stable states.

Migration as a source of insecurity is a much more recent phenomenon in the EU. It appeared after the Cold War and developed with the expansion of the EU towards Central and Eastern Europe (towards the communist states with issues in sticking to human and minority rights). Nowadays, against the intensification of the economic crisis, we are witnessing a new wave of economic migration (especially labour force) from the states of Central and Eastern Europe (much more affected by this phenomenon) to the developed ones in Western Europe. The immigrants have turned from invited-workers (in the reconstruction of European economies affected by World War II) into unwanted, second-class citizens, a burden to the welfare status of the social system, strongly affected by the economic crisis.

This wave gave rise to what is called "the fear of immigrants," a powerful tool in the hands of policymakers in times of economic crisis or an election campaign theme (see the case of the presidential campaign in France 2012 or the case of the parliamentary election campaign in Germany, 2003). Common threats are rearranged in "a spiral of insecurity" which culminates with the "image of the immigrant" perceived as "a nexus of all fears" (Arădău 2001, 3). Only in the twenty-first century (after the 2001 terrorist attacks), when immigration began to be seen as a combination of threats to the physical security of the state and social identity, does it firmly become incorporated into a "security continuum" (Ibid., 1).

After the 2001 terrorist attacks in the U.S. and their aftermath in Europe (Madrid 2004 and London 2005), the securitization of migration was achieved at an accelerated pace, being connected to certain recurrent themes on the international agenda such as organized crime, illegal activities, terrorism, and threats to identity and economic development. Security specialists strive to create an artificial connection between different activity sectors and uncontrolled migrations to justify the need for state intervention.

The disappearance of the external enemy determined the invention of an enemy within (the immigrant or the terrorist, for example), more difficult to identify and fought through asymmetric confrontation conditions, of low intensity and with ample reverberations in international security.

Hence, in the public discourse (of securitization), the migrant is presented as a threat to the internal labour market, the public order, cultural identity, economic development or solidarity. Huysmans argues that in this context migration is perceived as a threat to Western society: “Migration is identified as being one of the main factors weakening national tradition and societal homogeneity. It is reified as an internal and external danger for the survival of the national community or western civilization” (Huysman 2000, 758).

The same author considers that a neutral position in this matter is not possible, the two probable options being pro or con. In such conditions, supporting the immigration phenomenon is perceived as a threat to Western society values:

> This discourse excludes migrants from the normal fabric of society, not just as aliens but as aliens who are dangerous to the reproduction of the social fabric. The discourse frames the key question about the future of the political community as one of a choice for or against migration. But it is not a free choice because a choice for migration is represented as a choice against (the survival of) the political community. (Ibid.)

This positioning, based on Carl Schmitt’s theory (friend vs. enemy), condemns the immigrant to remain the source of insecurity, “the other,” the stranger. The former boundaries between the internal and external politics become ambiguous and the enemy or the previously well-defined threat are replaced by an infinity of dangerous beings/situations, causing Dillon to state that:

> Nothing is integrally safe and everything is integrally dangerous in this composite of (dis)order. There can, for example, be no single or simple state of emergency, no secure differentiation of self from other or friend from enemy, every self is an emergent self, every assemblage an emergent assemblage. (Dillon 2003)

Migration, as a source of insecurity, is a leitmotiv during the crisis period (particularly economic, which draws the limits of the welfare status) in the discourse of policymakers who justify their failure by finding “scapegoats” in the others, especially immigrants:

> The discourse reproduces the political myth that a homogenous national community or western civilization existed in the past and can be re-established today through the exclusion of those migrants who are identified as cultural aliens. (Huysman 2000, 758)

This is the case of the Roma who, although they are not a threat to the continent's security, as long as their socio-economic integration causes no major unbalances within the states they reside, with effects on the social and national security, are used as "scapegoats" in a series of violent events, like organized crime particularly against the person and personal property, street violence, and improvised dwellings on the outskirts of large cities (see the Mailat case in Italy 2008, Northern Ireland 2009 and France 2010–2012). The contextualization of these events to the economic crisis effects (the crisis of jobs, long-term unemployment, the housing crisis, the suppression of social benefits), all presented ostensibly by the media, gives rise to a real insecurity spiral.

The effects of this "media war" on an ethnic minority facing severe economic and social integration issues has allowed for "the transformation of a social issue into a problem of national security" (Iov 2012, 266), as evident in the Speech of Grenoble (2011) of Nicolas Sarkozy, the former president of France: "We must abolish the illegal Roma camps. These are areas where there is no right and that cannot be tolerated in France" (videos.tf1.fr). Moreover, this situation was also used to distract the French citizens' attention from the real social, economic and political problems of France (at that time), namely the reforming of the pension system, the job crisis or the Bettencourt corruption scandal (Evenimentul Zilei). The securitization process of the Roma issue in France allows for a multifaceted approach to the migration issue in the EU from the perspective of all the actors involved: the state of origin (social and economic issues determining migration), the transit states, the host state (national, identity, welfare status security), the media, the immigrants (social, economic and identity issues), the majority population in the host state, the civil society, and the EU as a desecuritization actor.

This complex network, and the implications of the migration phenomenon in a European Union that aims to become a political project, demonstrate the intricacy of this phenomenon, both as a study object for academia and as a politico-social concern for policymakers. From a historical point of view, the control over the immigration phenomenon is practically impossible in a European Union based on the free movement of persons, goods, products and services, European identity, and economic/single market liberalization, which require friendly borders.

Within the EU, there is a constant concern for the regularization of international migration, given that it decisively influences the economic development on the one hand (through migration of the cheap labour force and the migration of "brains/intelligence"), but at the same time, a total control over this phenomenon (in the sense of "zero migration") is unwanted and unattainable for economic and social development.

The enhancement of the cross-border cooperation and the creation of a European monitoring and control network (such as the Clubs of Berne and Wien, EUROPOL, FRONTEX, the GROTIUS programme) have led Bigo to speak of "a police archipelago" (reminiscent of Soljenytsin's Gulag Archipelago) (Arădău 2001, 5), mobilized by the EU to ensure a secure environment within the union. Unfortunately, this excessive securitization does not entail more security but draws attention to the immigration phenomenon in terms of increased illegal immigration, institutional incapacity and excessive securitization, leading to the idea of a "Fortress Europe."

The exacerbation of the migration phenomenon in the EU, particularly following the accession of Central and Eastern European states, has triggered xenophobia and intolerance, causing a sociological perspective on the migration security policy of "a Western Europe under siege" (Mamadouh 2012, 392) from immigrants.

Identity is a source of the sense and experience of individuals (Stivachtis 2008, 7), which cannot be defined unless related to the others, which individualizes and gives meaning to the existence of a group independent of its size or history. Identity is not a given, it is a social process, an intersubjective construct based on lived history, culture and the common language whose first word is "we," the second "us" with "them" being only the third (Castells 2004, 56) (in the sense of the others).

The relationship identity-security brings to the fore the multiple identities issue (that an individual acquires during their existence, some being more pronounced than others). From a liberal perspective, the only fundamental identity is derived from the nexus to the human race, with all other, secondary, identities (which are no less important) deriving from free will or tributary to the relationship with other individuals (acquired identity, in the sense of alterity). In another train of thought, for constructivists identity is constructed, is an ongoing process and not a given "exogenously to the human nature or internal policies systems" (Wendt 1994, 385).

The securitization of identity does not automatically imply a state of security for the host state's society, but rather leads to the emergence and supply of a state of insecurity (the dilemma of societal security). One possible answer to this state of insecurity is the multiculturalism policy promoted by the EU institutions (as desecuritization actors), starting with the motto "Unity in diversity!" (where diversity refers to the identities of various member states, which are replenished, as a corollary, by the European identity/European citizenship). Interculturality provides us with an interesting lesson of "transnational philosophy" (Liegeois 2008, 262). In the case of the European Union, the Roma are the centre of a multicultural project "that the Member States strive to manage" (Ibid.).

Multiculturalism, as a fundamental principle of the EU, brings to the fore the union's role as migration desecuritization actor (given that the free movement of persons, goods, services and capital underlie the EU construction). An important part is taken by the relationship European identity-national identity, both bringing into discussion the issue of imaged community. The European identity political project of building European citizenship gives coherence to the project of founding "The United States of Europe" (Ivan 2009) to complete the four fundamental liberties underlying the union.

The analysis focuses on demonstrating that migration goes beyond discursive practices, being an integral part of a complex construct, named the "security continuum" by Arădău. In this context, migration has been elevated to the level of meta-issue (Bigo 2001, 121–122), regarded as a spill-over effect, bringing together previous sectors of analysis that were studied separately and actors from different fields (from policymakers, to civil society and the media) with the hope of identifying viable solutions tailored to the causality relation migration-identity-(in)security in the EU. Given that immigration cannot be stopped (and "zero migration" is neither feasible nor desirable as it may have disastrous effects on economic and social development), and border control is illusory (Arădău 2001, 5), the threat to society is perpetual and inevitable (Ibid.).

The last two waves of accession consisting in states with a significant number of Roma populations living in precarious conditions tested the EU's integration ability. These two expansions were different from the previous ones both through the large number of applicants, history and the size of the population or the conflicts between the majority and the minority populations.

The European integration process in this case worked as a security system, determining a relocation of the state's role in terms of identity and sovereignty. European identity and citizenship are the centre of the integration process in recent years, within the wider debate on expansion vs. European integration. This debate has brought the democratic deficit the Union "suffers from" to the fore, and to which the Treaty of Lisbon has attempted to provide a possible solution adapted to the new requirements and challenges on the European agenda.

Security has always been the purpose behind the European integration process, in an attempt of the states to securitize the mistakes of the twentieth century. Since the beginning of the 1960s, a series of transformations have affected the European Community, and after the Maastricht Treaty the primarily economic community fell into a political union track in an attempt to become "The United States of Europe" (Ivan 2009).

Building the Europe of tomorrow cannot be achieved without a consensus regarding international migration and its medium- or long-term effects on security, social cohesion, the welfare state and identity in the EU. In this context, the EU Member States (attractive to immigrants due to the social protection system or economic opportunities) have shown constant concern in perfecting the legislation on migration.

Identity innovates the migration-insecurity causality relation, conferring it flexibility and referential value both at a sub- and supranational level, giving rise to a trans-disciplinary research agenda.

References

Arădău, C. (2001). Migration: The Spiral of (In)Security, *International Forum of Electronic Publications*. Online: http://web.archive.org/web/20070403192142/http://venus.ci.uw.edu.pl/~rubikon/forum/claudia1.html.

Bigo, D. (2001). Migration and Security. In V. Guiraudon & C. Joppke (Eds.), *Controlling a New Migration World*. London: Routledge.

Castells, M. (2004). *The power of Identity*. London: Blackwell.

Choucri, N. (2002). Migration and Security: Some Key Linkages. *Journal of International Affairs 56 (1)*: 98-122.

Dillon, M. (2003). Virtual Security: A Life Science of (Dis)Order. *Millenium 32 (3)*: 531-558.

Huysmans, J. (2000). The European Union and the Securitization of Migration. *Journal of Common Market Studies 38 (5)*: 751-777.

Iov, C. A. (2012). Situaţia romilor în Uniunea Europeană între ignoranţa şi repatriere: Cazul Franţei [The Roma situation in the European Union between ignorance and repatriation: The Case of France]. *Simpozionul Internaţional "Universul Ştiinţelor,"* Iaşi: Pim PH. 266-268.

Ivan, A. (2009). *Sub zodia "Statelor Unite ale Europei." De la idea europeană la Comunităţile Economice Europene* [Under the sign of the "United States of Europe": From the European idea to the European Economic Communities]. Cluj-Napoca: C & A Publishing.

Liegeois, J. P. (2008). *Romii în Europa* [The Roma in Europe]. Bucureşti: Monitorul Oficial.

Mamadouh, V. (2012). The Scaling of the 'Invasion', A Geopolitics of Immigration Narratives in France and The Netherlands. *Geopolitics 17 (2)*: 377-401. Online: http://dx.doi.org/10.1080/14650045.2011.578268.

Sarcinschi, A. (2008). *Migraţie şi Securitate* [Migration and Security] Bucureşti: Editura Universităţii Naţionale de Apărare "Carol I." Online: http://cssas.unap.ro/ro/pdf_studii/migratie_si_securitate.pdf.

Sarkozy, N. (2010). *Discours a Grenoble*. Online: http://videos.tf1.fr/infos/2010/le-discours-de-nicolas-sarkozy-a-grenoble-dans-son-integralite-5953237.html.

Scandal in Franţa: puterea spionează ziariştii [Scandal in France: the power is spying on the journalists]. Evenimentul Zilei, 9 decembrie 2011. Online: http://www.evz.ro/detalii/stiri/scandal-in-franta-puterea-spioneaza-ziaristii-943976.html.

Stivachtis, Y. A. (2008). International Migration and the Politics of Identity and Security. *Journal of Humanities and Social Science 2 (1)*. Online: http://www.scientificjournals.org/journals2008/articles/1387.pdf.

Wendt, A. (1994). Collective Identity formation and the International State. *American Political Science Review 88*: 384-396.

MOBILIZING YOUTH ON SOCIALIST CONSTRUCTION SITES AND REDEFINING IDENTITY

DANIELA-MIHAELA SPÎNU-DUMITRU

Introduction

Communist industrialization and urbanization bring concepts such as new lives, new paths, internal migration, fighting or work to the forefront. In the centre of these ideological borders we rediscover the youth as "the most interesting part of human society because they are the future, which is born and develops in society, the citizens of tomorrow" (*Scînteia* June 27, 1948).

Moreover, the Central Committee of the Romanian Communist Party stated in messianic terms, at the Unification Congress of Youth Organization in 1948, the role of youth in building socialism: "they must be at the forefront in the struggle for the fulfilment of the socialist reorganization of the state" (*Scînteia* June 7, 1948)

Resita, Hunedoara, Cluj, Targu Mures, Brasov or Galati are some of the cities that became sites of socialist construction (*Scînteia* July 21, 1949).

Seen through the ideological lens, these spaces become sites of inoculation of new principles of life, where "the future citizen is born, which should give new cohorts of conscious people, full of enthusiasm" (*Scînteia* May 23, 1948). While being "an epic battle showing how participation in that battle transfigured the individual making him a true socialist" (Lenoe 2004, 213), the construction site, as a place of migration, promoted transformative power, pretending to be an apparatus by which "fearful, passive, insecure village labourers would be transformed into class conscious, fighting workers" (Pittaway 2012, 7).

"Eaglets of plants and lands" (*Scînteia* June 7, 1948), as the young were about to be called on the great national sites, became the artefacts of a new life.

In this context, our chapter aims are to allot, by following the ideological pattern, the role of socialist construction sites in the reconstruction of youth identity.

Methods

This chapter focuses on the discourse and content analysis of the socialist propaganda of the *Scînteia* newspaper, bringing together articles between 1948 and 1950. The selected period includes the most effervescent stage regarding the regime's attempt to promote patterns of behaviour for the so-called "new people."

The use of these sources stands for an essential benchmark even more as Raymond Bauer & David Gleicher (1953, 297) maintain that: "the regime attempts not only to determine what information and ideas shall pass through the media, but also who shall have access to what information and ideas."

Certainly, it would be interesting to see if this ideological policy found its correspondent in real life and to what extent individuals identified with it.

Discussion

The Political Report of CC (The Central Committee) presented by Gheorghe Gheorghiu Dej to the National Conference of PCR (*Scînteia* November 1, 1945) from 1945 brought the issue of the conversion of the war industries to the forefront. The report text underlined:

> … this transition should not be left only to private isolated initiatives. The new production of these enterprises must be guided on the essential needs connected to the economic recovery of the country, based on plans drawn up for each branch and taking into account not only the production capacity, but also the kind and extent of the internal needs and of the existing import and export possibilities. (*Scînteia* November 1, 1945)

In this respect, the Soviet examples demonstrate that:

> some factories moved to the manufacturing of lightweight tourist bikes; other factories moved to the repetitive work of refrigerated cabinets and gas corks. There is also the repetitive work of beds, dishes, meat grinders, spoons, thermometers, teapots, door locks, prams and sleighs. There are also factories preparing for manufacturing farming machinery, combine harvesters, croppers, milling facilities and engines for farming machinery.

> Other factories are to manufacture buses, boats, electric train engines and electric installations for mines. (*Scinteia* November 1, 1945)

"The years of building on a large scale," as it was to be called later, metaphorically speaking, through state industrialization produce the image of sites and factories whose main actor becomes the young worker, the prototype of the new man.

"Come, you too, on the site"—*Scînteia* and the Mobilization of the Youth

"The entire site is preparing to welcome its bricklayers. The bedrooms are clean and nicely decorated. Inside the workshops the turners and the carpenters are creating dozens of tanks" (*Scînteia*, March 22, 1950). Petre Modrog wrote home to the lads of the village that "Here there is more and more to work and the site is expanding. Come you too, to build together!" (*Scînteia* March 22, 1950). Focussing on the site conditions, the above quotation represents one of the most eloquent examples of instigation to migration.

In addition, due to the fact that labour was voluntary, a series of symbolic stories were promoted:

> A brigade of Magyars from Alba Iulia came. They were poor youth, unemployed. A malevolent had told the young that they would get all kind of gifts for their labour and until they came to the site, some of them started to believe that. The night when they came and were told bluntly that the young are called to be volunteers, without other special benefits, some wanted to go back. When the sector commander wanted to give them the return roadmaps, the youth brigades from the barracks came together. Then the sector commander told everyone: some young people from the Alba Iulia brigade are leaving the site since here we have voluntary work. The girls of the others blushed. The young man Mogos came of their midst forward and really blushed and his eyes wet stared into the ground, said in a low voice: Well then, I have never been so ashamed before in my life! (*Scînteia* April 12, 1948)

Voluntary work implies ambition, courage, power of sacrifice, and the defining elements of the new man "who looks with love at his work knowing that its outgrowth is in his own benefit" (*Scînteia* April 12, 1948).

Therewith, voluntary work remains the passport to an apprentice position in the new plants. The construction industry, sustains Kenneth Straus (1997, 106), was to become a conveyer belt "providing the peasant recruits with the experience that would prepare them to deal with the factory system and urban life. Once a new factory was built, the factory administration would generally attempt to keep the construction workers and put them to work in production" (Ibid.)

First the site, and then the factory, far from being a place of exploitation, as in capitalism, it became a "work place managed by skilled, literate and dutiful workmen, proud of their labour" (Kotkin 1995, 203).

Although the articles do not hesitate to use adjectives such as "hard," "difficult" or "exhausting," the benefits do not delay to arise: "work is not easy, but people work impetuously and enthusiastically. The mirror of how impetuously they work represents the honour board placed at the site entrance and on which are registered the names of those who showed off" (*Scînteia* September 23, 1949).

The detail is extremely interesting, in so far as the individuals build their identity in relation to their workplace and their name, failing to define the job, becoming a chain of characters.

The youth transform the site and the site transforms the youth

The communist industrialization led to the generating of some fundamental rapture (Ianoş 2008) in the city structure not only regarding the internal macrostructure, but also its physiognomy. Moreover, as a series of sociologic analyses suggests, the industrialization led to creating a real "social psychology of migrations" (Constantinescu, Stahl & Drăgan 1974, 60), especially among the young.

However, the migrants from the Soviet period were considered "a mass of people that were wandering, without a precise goal, without any plan," being in a ceaseless mobility labelled "Brownian, chaotic, involving a series of real effects" (Ibid., 29).

In this context, the internal migration as a social process is not transposed in terms of an urbanization, but mainly as a "deruralization" which transforms the individuals in an intermediary social class, nor as peasants, in that the deruralization process implies the abandon of a traditional way of life, nor townsmen.

The evolution of urban society is perceived as directly dependent on the evolution of an urban environment, the newly created society wearing the "footprint of the socialist action, becoming more and more its product" (Ibid., 126).

Following this particularity, the transforming role of communist industrialization and urbanization is felt in the capacity of creation and development of "a way of life open to new and fast transformations" (Ibid., 126).

The complexity of urbanization evoked by Lewin (2003) refers to a series of essential changes felt by the mobile population.

Leaving the traditional rural communities, the contact with "the world of sites and cities," with various individuals, imposes the rethinking of one's own identity:

> … the ideas that flow through the new means of communication, expose the population to a flood of information, creating new concepts on existence and new personal needs … the newcomer finds himself exposed, to his amazement, to a huge variety of beliefs, personalities, ways of dressing, information, values that affect ceaselessly the social, family and traditional spaces. (Ibid., 400)

Considering these reasons, the communist newspaper *Scînteia*, as an ideological extension of PCR, imposes the guidelines that must be followed to transform the youth. Redefining identity must not be a process left to chance, but must be guided by clear rules, by default, since where the work lacks perspective the individuals "first get covered with mould, then they turn grey, afterwards they are overwhelmed by the swamp of daily needs, finally transforming into the most common citizens" (*Scînteia* May 23, 1949).

The young workers must be directed towards self study, culture, the cultural programs and manifestations being conceived "not as a simple party, but in connection with the site matters" (*Scînteia* May 23, 1948).

Moreover, it was required that the site, a "huge laboratory under the open sky" (*Scînteia* June 8, 1950), should provide the "fight for raising the level and tailoring a new path in life" (*Scînteia* May 27, 1948).

Collective work, the competitions between brigades, sectors, sites, the exchange of experience between workmen, as well as the agitators' activities, became emergent factors of change: "they must be aware that what they have learnt as good and useful on the site, that the change happened inside themselves, the gaining of self-confidence, of their strengths and abilities, the determination that arose to look bravely at the hardships, all of these are due to the Party" (*Scînteia* May 23, 1948).

Forthwith, the first proofs of "change" are recorded in the newspaper: "when the first school for illiterates was open, the youth from the brigades gave up their cigarettes which they sold in order to buy notebooks and pencils for the school students" (*Scînteia* May 15, 1948).

The more the plant grows, the better people grow stories about the new people

The promoted strategy through the *Scînteia* newspaper reflects the regime trial to transform the various workmen from various social categories into townsmen, to level them, and especially, in a radically changed social framework, to induce their integration.

Within this context, the new man develops in the young workers, volunteers of the site:

> … he grows when he climbs the rocky cliffs, when he creeps through pools through the holes of the tunnel, when he fixes new work standards which he overcomes, when he pulls down the haughty crests of the mountains, when he fills with rocks the wild steeps. The new man, the new young person who is singing while working, whose eyes gleam while working. The workman, who gathers and collects, unites and guides the others towards the same lofty ideals. (*Scînteia* April 12, 1948)

Young, unmarried, with a limited life experience, the new Soviet man "crosses frontiers and breaks barriers of mentalities" (Chambers 1994, 2). Sharing the living space, deprived of intimacy, between two worlds, the young workmen become, Chambers maintains, the ideal category to inoculate the belief of building socialism at a time when the only safety landmark is the party alone.

Certainly, the examples of those that wish to venture into building socialism, becoming what Sheila Fitzpatrick (1999, 74) calls "ordinary celebrities" or "celebrities for a day," do not cease to rise; firstly those from USSR, then those at the national level.

Stepan Golovkin, a mechanic at the bearing plant from Moscow, tells how his life changed after the site experience:

> I was born in Galkino village which belongs nowadays to the Kalinin region. My mother was illiterate, and my father could hardly read and write. During the Soviet regime my life changed entirely. In those days there was the end of fitting installations at the bearing plant. At the same time the workmen who were about to work at the new machinery were trained. This plant became my destiny; all my family joys are tied to it. The plant gave me a flat in a new building, in the beautiful working class town that was built around the plant. Right from the first days I started to learn, I graduated the foremen school, and then the courses for the technical staff, I acquired knowledge equivalent to those they teach you at the technical middle school. (*Scînteia* April 13, 1950)

At Resita, Radu Nicolac, was appointed team leader, and Dragota Chifor became craftsman from plain worker (*Scînteia* April 1, 1950). At Hunedoara, Ion Simionov, born in a fishing family from Tulcea, "came on site when the first brigadiers' barracks were built. At the beginning he worked with the shovel and the pickaxe, then he followed the qualification school I and II and this day he is a skilled electrician" (*Scînteia* March 13, 1950). The same happened in Fagaras: "when he came to the site plant, Grigore Smeu was a plain mechanic. Today he is chief foreman of the central workshop. Raised and educated by the Party, he always stepped resolutely forward, overcoming the hardships that kept coming" (*Scînteia* March 16, 1950). And such examples may go on.

The rebirth of man and society on the whole stopped being a utopian project, becoming true through the life stories of some common people who succeeded in transforming themselves through work and culture.

Results

The construction site is not just a space for physical labour, but a real laboratory in which the young are redefining their identity through "increasing self-confidence, strength and capacity, enduring bravely the hardships" (*Scînteia* May 23, 1948). Moreover, through the proliferation of cultural and artistic manifestations "still not as a mere party but linked to sites issues" by "stimulating cultural thirst" (*Scînteia* June 27, 1948), the publication reiterates the real values that should underpin the next generation, the construction site functioning as a launch pad into adult life.

Disposing phrases like "when he came he was more secluded. He didn't attend any UTM school, was not activist and now he is a technical manager" (*Scînteia* June 9, 1948), or "comrade Vasiliu today is no longer a simple brigadier, today he is a young firm worker, cultural responsible with the whole sector of the construction site," *Scînteia* translates the work experience on the construction site as a process of maturation and identity reconfiguration, the leitmotif being their responsibility "for the fate of their country, for the victory of socialist construction" (Pittaway 2012, 7).

References

Bauer, R. & Gleicher, D. (1953). Word-of-Mouth Communication in the Soviet Union. *Public Opinion Quarterly 17*: 297-310.

Chambers, I. (1994). *Migrancy, Culture and Identity*. New York, NY: Routledge.

Constantinescu, M., Stahl, H. H. & Drăgan, I. (1974). *Le processus d'urbanisation en Roumanie*. Bucharest : Meridiane.
Fitzpatrick, S. (1999). *Everyday Stalinism: Ordinary Life in Extraordinary Times: Soviet Russia in the 1930's*. Oxford: Oxford University Press.
Ianoş, I. (2008). A major challenge for Romanian towns. The "large habitats". In G. Pomeroy & G. Webster (Eds.), *Global Perspective on Globalization*. Lanham, MD: University Press of America. 106-135.
Kotkin, S. (1997). *Magnetic Mountain: Stalinism as a Civilization*. Berkeley, CA: University of California Press.
Lenoe, M. (2004). *Closer to the Masses: Stalinist Culture, Social Revolution, and Soviet Newspapers*. Cambridge, MA: Harvard University Press.
Lewin, M. (2003). *Le siècle soviétique* [The Soviet Century]. Paris: Fayard.
Pittaway, M. (2012). *The Workers' State: Industrial Labor and the Making of Socialist Hungary, 1944-1958*. Pittsburgh: University of Pittsburgh Press.
Scînteia, May 27, 1949
—. April 1, 1950
—. April 12, 1948
—. April 13, 1950
—. July 21, 1949
—. June 27, 1948
—. June 7, 1948
—. June 7, 1948
—. June 8, 1950
—. June 9, 1948
—. March 13, 1950
—. March 16, 1950
—. March 22, 1950
—. May 15, 1948
—. May 23, 1948
—. May 27, 1948
—. November 1, 1945
—. September 23, 1949
Straus, K. (1997). *Factory and Community in Stalin's Russia: The Making of an Industrial working class*. Pittsburgh: University of Pittsburgh Press.

REINTEGRATING VULNERABLE IMMIGRANT GROUPS ON THE LABOUR MARKET

LAVINIA-ELISABETA POPP AND FELICIA ANDRIONI

Introduction

Employment in the period of transition to the market economy in Romania is a very important issue, with connotations determined by the fact that it takes place on an imperfect labour market, rigid, segmented, fragile, demographically aged and dominated by massive emigration. Under these circumstances, the restructuring of the Romanian social-economic system, in accordance with the market economy requirements, triggered deep changes on the Romanian labour market and led to the occurrence of unemployment as a mass phenomenon, and generated strong impediments which limited access to the labour market for the vulnerable immigrant groups (i.e. old people, young people, women, rural inhabitants, and persons with low levels of education and training).

The term "vulnerable group" is often used in official documents, legislative documents or in research reports as similar to disadvantaged, marginalised, excluded or at-risk groups, all these concepts being related to the wider phenomenon of poverty (Popescu 2011). In order to identify vulnerable groups social-demographic features such as gender, age, ethnic origin, geographic location, education, occupation, etc. are used. The individual lives in a world of economic, spiritual, legal and political values concomitantly with the world of social groupings (Georgevici 2013).

Methods and Techniques

Data Source. The approach is represented by a comparative study regarding the opportunities of reintegration for vulnerable groups to the labour market in Caraş-Severin and Hunedoara counties. The comparative analysis aims, on the one hand, at enriching the set of information related to the reintegration modalities in which vulnerable immigrant groups can be integrated into the labour market, and on the other at identifying the factors underlying a qualified labour force, adapted to the market requirements, by ensuring positive correlations between the skills supply and the labour market demand. This research responds to the need for collecting information and elaborating policies on a subject that has not been sufficiently studied in the literature. Furthermore, it falls within the preoccupations of authorities to integrate the vulnerable immigrant population in the labour market.

The **Study Purpose** is to enhance the degree of awareness regarding the immigration phenomenon in Romania and to support the social integration of vulnerable immigrant groups (old and young people, women, rural inhabitants, persons with low levels of education and qualifications) in the Caraş-Severin and Hunedoara counties, and elaborate a diagnosis of the current situation related to the situation of foreigners in the two counties, as well as the population's perception of foreigners and their integration into Romanian society

Research Objectives

- Conduct an analysis about the effects of professional training programmes on the main components of the labour market in the two counties subjected to the survey
- Analysis of causes triggering a poor performance on the labour market, in relation to the immigrant vulnerable groups, contributing to poverty, inequality and social exclusion in the context of the present social-economic policies
- Identification of factors ensuring a qualified immigrant labour force as well as provision of a positive correlation between the supply of skills and demand on the labour market.

The target group is represented by the population of foreigners in the Mountain Banat and Jiu Valley areas, the public institutions in charge of the two counties, as well as non-governmental organisations involved in the management of immigration and integration of vulnerable immigrant persons. The respondents were selected through the random method, which allows for the possibility of analysing the general perceptions of the entire population and changes occurring as a result of the immigrants' presence within the community.

Research Questions

- What are the significant elements of the employment policies leaving a positive mark or negatively influencing immigrant employment in the two regions' communities?
- To what extent do social, economic, health and educational policies influence the poor performances of vulnerable immigrant groups on the labour market in Caraş Severin and Hunedoara counties?

Methodology

Methodological clarifications. The methodological dimensions related to the opportunities of vulnerable immigrant groups' integration to the labour market suppose a combination between the normative and interpretative analysis of the data collected. The normative approach starts from the description of the phenomenon under study by using the semi-structured interview and the sociological questionnaire. The interpretative approach starts from the analysis of the social phenomenon "as such," reflected in social reality by means of observation. Different data result from the two types of analysis, as the normative analysis is focused on what is explainable, verifiable, quantifiable, objective and external in reality, whereas the second interpretation mostly analyses what is interpretative, subjective, unique and internal (Cohen & Manion 1981, in Demazière 1996). These investigative methods intend to contribute to the comprehension and explanation of social reality from two different angles: the normative analysis starts from the idea that the general-normative laws determine the individual's social and professional behaviour, while the interpretative one analyses the data collected from the operational perspective, based on the individual's interactions.

The design of the methodological research was structured in the following stages:

- The preliminary theoretical stage represented by the documentary office research, and the documentation endeavour supposed a process of collecting relevant information and statistic data, analyses of public institutions reports, consultation of quantitative and qualitative studies and researches focused on these topics, and informal discussions with representatives of non-governmental organisations or public institutions.

- The stage of data collecting, highlighted through the applied research, is illustrated by the methodology represented by semi-structured interviews, as well as the sociologic questionnaire. In order to select the respondents, indicators were used in the qualitative part of the research to significantly influence the perception, attitudes and behaviours of Romanian citizens toward foreigners (age, education level and belonging to a religious or ethnic group). A fifteen-minute, multi-themed questionnaire was applied, and the collection manner consisted of face-to-face interviews.
- Processing and interpretation of the collected quantitative and qualitative data.
- Completion of research and expected results. Among the most important results expected from the applied research we may list: a wider scope of information on the immigration phenomenon; raising awareness of the Caraş-Severin and Hunedoara population on the immigration phenomenon, for the reduction of social exclusion and discriminatory practices; enhancement of vulnerable immigrants' access to information regarding public services and programmes provided by the Romanian Office for Immigrations and other institutions and organisations, and an increase of authorities' capacity to offer integrated services to vulnerable immigrants, adapted to the existing realities.

During our investigative endeavour we analysed the similitudes and disparities of the distribution of a set of analysis indicators related to education and professional training which induce social-economic, demographic, technological and cultural challenges in the two counties (Caraş-Severin and Hunedoara) subjected to the survey, through the realisation, in the first stage of the exploratory analysis, of a complex descriptive profile of the disadvantaged groups on the one hand, and through the completion of an analysis focused on the effects produced by the professional training programmes on the main components of the local labour market on the other.

The research instruments utilised were: the semi-structured interview guide focused on the themes resulting from the discussions with the representatives of governmental institutions and non-governmental organisations active in the field of foreigners' integration in Caraş Severin and Hunedoara, as well as the sociological questionnaire, destined to the immigrant vulnerable groups; the data analysis grid; and the chart of the statistic and comparative indicators' analysis.

Measures. From the applied research it follows that in both Caraş Severin and Hunedoara counties, with insignificant variations, the analysis of the structure by genders and age groups of vulnerable immigrants (old people, youth, rural inhabitants, persons with a low level of education and qualification) points out that men represent 57%–58% of the total immigrants. However, in the 35–65 age range their proportion increases even more, and reaches the values of 68% for men and 28% for women. When analysing the distribution of immigrants by age groups, we remark that the immigrant population is a young population, active on the labour market, with productive potential. Moreover, the age structure of immigrants in Romania constitutes a premise and potential solution for Romania's demographic issue, as we are an ageing society with high emigration and a low birth rate (Alexe & Păunescu 2011). Nationally, the available statistical information related to the permanent immigration evolution allows us to better understand the dynamics of the immigrants' numbers and consequently the gender structure for immigration in the analysed counties. The immigrants' gender structure, according to the data provided by ORI, indicates an approximately equal gender distribution in 2000, but the women's percentage in the total number of immigrants has constantly decreased to reach a level below 40%, especially in recent years (Alexe & Păunescu 2011).

As regards foreigners with permanent residence, most come from Moldova, China and Turkey in both counties, but particularly in Hunedoara the low number of immigrants from the United States has exhibited greater dynamics in recent years.

Foreigners' integration in Caraş-Severin and Hunedoara counties is easier in big cities than in small towns or in the rural environment, is a process taking place in several stages, and the policies of the vision and practical implementation of integration need to follow the same path. In this respect, we may say that the integration process starts before arrival, and at the same time we may appreciate how important it is to adopt an integration policy focused on newcomers. Social networks based on relatives and friends provide support for the immigrants' settlement, for penetration of the new immigration environment, and adaptation to local conditions (Alexe & Păunescu 2011).

We may list the following issues, highlighted in both counties, that represent inhibiting factors during the integration route: constant change of required documents, postponements on the part of the institutions with which immigrants come in contact, documents that expire until new ones are released, clerks in public institutions with whom they interact not being aware of the rights and legislation applied to foreigners in Romania, and a shortage of qualified personnel.

A considerable number of respondents benefit from cultural orientation training, but we must underline the problems regarding this dimension, i.e. obstacles related to Romanian language courses and cultural orientation. The main domains in which vulnerable immigrants were employed in Caraş Severin are light industry and services (hotels, commerce, etc.) and in Hunedoara county construction and services. They are usually employed by firms owned by their fellow countrymen. In many cases, the bare necessities, such as housing, subsistence means, etc. are facilitated by the communities of immigrants to which they belong, even if employers only occasionally offer them some facilities (e.g. housing, transport, or meals).

Data Analysis. All analyses were performed using SPSS 15 for Microsoft Windows. Given the exploratory purposes of the study, only descriptive statistics was computed.

Results

The recommendations based on the finding of facts and desires expressed by the interviewed or questioned respondents referred to: the improvement of access to the Romanian language and cultural orientation courses (as immigrants ignore the offer, do not know who offers the training or what steps to take to enrol in Romanian language training courses, they encounter logistic difficulties in organisation and material resources allotment); adaptation of the course schedules to working hours, as well as the necessity of using modern teaching methods and materials so that the rapid learning of the language can be facilitated; offering certificates on the completion of courses attesting the language knowledge level, and the supply of Romanian courses should include both initiation and advanced or improvement of language courses.

In general, the persons immigrating in the two counties subjected to the study do it for employment or commercial activities. Most immigrants are men, aged between 35 and 45, married, with one or two small children, and in general do not wish to attend professional courses or other forms of training. Few of them travel outside Romania (depending on material possibilities, distance to the origin country or family situation). The highest mobility is found in the Turkish and Moldovan communities whose citizens travel to their origin countries at least once a year. Immigrants' involvement in the life of Romanian society is reduced. In their spare time, immigrants go to their fellow countrymen's circles (e.g.

restaurants, places of worship), attend their national cultural events, or meet with small groups of Romanian friends. Up to the present, the media has seldom approached the issues of vulnerable immigrants in Romania.

Barriers. Some terminological and utilisation obstacles encountered were confusion related to the terms "migrant," "immigrant," "refugees," "asylum applicant"; the reorganisation of the institutional system often leads to modifications of the data collected in the domain of immigration and foreigners' integration; there are very few statistic data calculated for the immigrants in the areas of social, economic, cultural and educational integration, or civic participation (Alexe & Păunescu 2011)

Discussion and Conclusions

The study, although containing an important explanatory side, does not aim at providing a complete answer to the existing questions related to the employment of vulnerable groups. In this respect it is necessary to have very detailed knowledge of the problems generated by employment, unemployment, and normal operation of the labour market (elimination of dysfunctionalities, optimisation of relations) depending, in the present context, on a multitude of facts regarding the institutional and legislative reality.

The European policies regarding immigration still have an ambivalent and ambiguous character, undergoing a process of permanent transformation and adaptation. The EU community and national legislation constitute on the one hand agents of exchange, and on the other a source of controversy and misunderstanding.

As for the integration capacity of immigrant groups in Romania, children, students and businesspersons have the highest potential. The problems in this sense are raised by the persons in their care or the vulnerable groups such as women and old people. Men are more active than women in the social, cultural and economic life of Romanian society due to the traditional role within the family, and to the cultural and religious features (Alexe, Popescu & Toth 2009).

In the process of the integration of vulnerable immigrant persons into Romanian society the following recommendations are important: improving communication with public authorities, both centrally and locally, and with the Romania population; creating opportunities for the improvement of skills, supply of counselling services, support for vulnerable persons on the labour market; adopting solutions for adjustment, special social care, medical care, psychological treatment, etc.; treating children, women, old persons and other disadvantaged persons in an undiscriminating manner; and developing measures meant to promote the involvement of women and old people in the social, economic and cultural life of society.

References

Alexe, I. & Păunescu, B. (Eds.). (2011). *Study on the immigration phenomenon in Romania. Aliens' integration into the Romanian society*. Online: http://ec.europa.eu/ewsi/en/resources/detail.cfm?ID_ITEMS=20205.

Alexe, I., Popescu, R &.Toth, G. (2009). Research report: Immigrants' information needs in Romania. Bucureşti: Fundaţia Soros.

Demazière, D. (1996). Experienţa şomajului în Franţa: procese de excludere şi construcţia identităţii [Experiencing Unemployment in France: Exclusion Processes and Identity Construction]. In A. Neculau & G. Ferreol (Eds.), *Minoritari, marginali, excluşi*. Iaşi: Polirom. 191-194.

European Fund for the Integration of Third Country Nationals 2007-2013. Online: http://www.unife.it/ricerca/finanziamenti-gestione/ricerca-internazionale/Bando%20Immigrati%202007.pdf.

Georgevici, G. F. (2013). Monographic Sociology of Dimitrie Gusti. Social Science and Reform. *European University Studies, Sociology, XXII (454)*: 1-123.

Popescu, R. (2011). *Vulnerable groups and social economy. Rroma ethnics and women in difficulty. Intervention Manual*. Bucureşti: Expert.

USE OF LANGUAGE LEARNING STRATEGIES BY RETIRED BRITISH PEOPLE IN NON-ENGLISH SPEAKING COUNTRIES

AMADOR JIMÉNEZ-GARRIDO
AND EUFRASIO PEREZ-NAVIO

Introduction

"Displacement has become the most powerful imagery for the modern world" (Anthias 2006, 17). Spain is the preferred destination for UK retirees. The increasing amount of elderly foreigners that choose the Costa del Sol as their retirement destination has caught the attention of many researchers interested in not just the reasons for this migration but the characteristics of this twenty-first century occurrence.

Retiring abroad is a common strategy used by aged people to make the best of the last part of their lives (King, Warnes & Williams 1998), and the desire for a better leisure-oriented life combined with recreational and service resources often leads this decision (Rowles & Watkins 1993). The trigger for international retirement is mainly the traits of destination and the characteristic of the people who decide to take the step of moving abroad. Normally, the weather represents the main deciding factor for the destination country (Friedrich & Warnes 2000), and the previous experiences in the area by other country fellows are also important (Cuba & Longino 1991). The cost of living has a very strong impact in the final decision of living in another country. The housing market price is a determinant factor for the elderly as it is strongly related to the capacity of affording a more luxurious lifestyle. Glasgow (1995) mentions in his research that the permission to use health services is, in the long term, a paramount factor, as the age of the people involved in this migration phenomenon indicates that they are more likely to use it, and do so more frequently.

On the other hand, the language barrier is the main drawback. The inability to communicate with locals efficiently hinders networking outside the community of people of the same country of origin. Betty Cahill (1997) claims that the retired abroad show a lack of disposition to learn the local language, especially if they are English speakers. This language is considered the current *lingua franca* and its speakers expect and assume that it should be spoken almost everywhere, and at least in touristic locations. Hardill (2006) mentions that the lack of proficiency in the local language limits the integration of foreign retirees in the destination country. Only 25% of the British retirees on the Costa del Sol consider themselves proficient enough to maintain conversation with locals (Casado-Diaz, Kaiser & Warnes 2004). The advanced age of these circumstantial learners is a problem if we consider the theory of the Critical Period Hypotheses, which basically agrees that age is a factor in learning languages and that it comes in the "bioprogram" of each person, rather than thinking that language learning is set by environmental conditions (Birdsong 1999). Bornstein (1989, 179) defines the critical age for language learning as the time in the life cycle when many structures and functions become especially susceptible to specific experiences (or to the absence of those experiences) in a way that alters some future instantiation of that (or a related) structure or function. Following in the same line of thought, Newport (1991, 112) identifies: "any phenomenon in which there is a maturational change in the ability to learn, with a peak in learning at some maturationally definable period … and a decline in the ability to learn, given the same experiential exposure, outside of this period." In light of this worldwide accepted theory, the age of the retirees will be an important drawback in learning a second language and an important factor to pay attention to.

A lot has been said about the reasons for migration among European retirees in other countries. Nonetheless, the specific drawbacks of this movement are yet to be explored in depth. The purpose of this study is to see how the migrants cope with the local language obstacle and the dimension of the strategies used to make communication with locals more efficient and smooth. Secondly, as mentioned, the age of the migrants will be an important factor for analysis.

Methods and Techniques

Participants and geographical location of the study. A total of fifty-six retired British people agreed to complete the questionnaires of this study. The location chosen for participation was the Costa del Sol in Malaga, Spain, more specifically in the towns of Benalmadena and Torremolinos. These two settlements are conveniently located near the large-sized city

Malaga, which has an international airport that is very well connected to many other cities in Europe. Altogether, these aspects have created a favourite spot for British retires, who have created a large colony in turn. Participation in the study was conditioned by the status of retirees with a minimum of two years residence in the area. The difference between the concepts of tourist and resident are a little blurred and there is a great amount of doubt when asking a retired migrant about their situation in Spain. This inability to describe their conjecture in the country is derived from the length of the stay in the destination country and the social commitments with the local communities. In order to be eligible to take a resident permit in Spain, a person must have spent 183 days or more there. Anything below this mark legally represents a "retired long-term tourist," and the country of residence is somewhere other than Spain. For that reason, before answering any questionnaire the participants were asked if they were residents, or if they did not know their status they were asked if they spent more than six months per year in Spain. In addition, the study opted to consider subjects resident in the area for at least two years, but cumulatively rather than consecutively.

Procedure. A first questionnaire was created to gather information about the age of the participants and the length of their stay in the country, and no other personal information. The second questionnaire is version 7.0 of the "Strategy Inventory for Language Learning" (henceforth SILL), as created by Oxford in 1989. This is a fifty-item questionnaire that uses a Likert Scale in its answers, evaluating the frequency of use of language learning strategies by second language learners. The items of this questionnaire are divided into six categories: memory, cognitive, compensation, metacognitive, affective and social. This tool has been used worldwide for twenty years to describe how second language learners face the language barrier.

Several ideas were considered regarding the distribution of the questionnaires. The first one was to write a proposal to retiree clubs in the area. This idea was dismissed, as in general this sort of club or society brings together people with many similarities, which would have limited the scope of answers. The second option considered was to seek participants around the international airport of Malaga. Unfortunately, access to the gates as visitor was not granted. Third, it was thought that given the good time span and random distribution of British retirees along the beaches of Benalmadena it would be apposite to approach them when they are enjoying a sunny day near the sea. Another decision was to ask for the participation of one member of the same family only, as in the pilot collection procedure the answers found in members of the same family were meaningfully similar.

Discussion and Results

As has been said, the goal of this descriptive piece of research is to gather more details on how the British retirees cope with language from the point of view of the language learning strategies used or preferred. Age and length of the stay abroad are two important variables in this study. These two scale types of variables will be grouped in five-year ranges for the age of the participants and two-year ranges for the length of stay.

Figure 2-1 below shows the number of participants per age range. Retirees between 65 and 70 have the most participants with 23. Ten participants are more than 70 and less than 75.

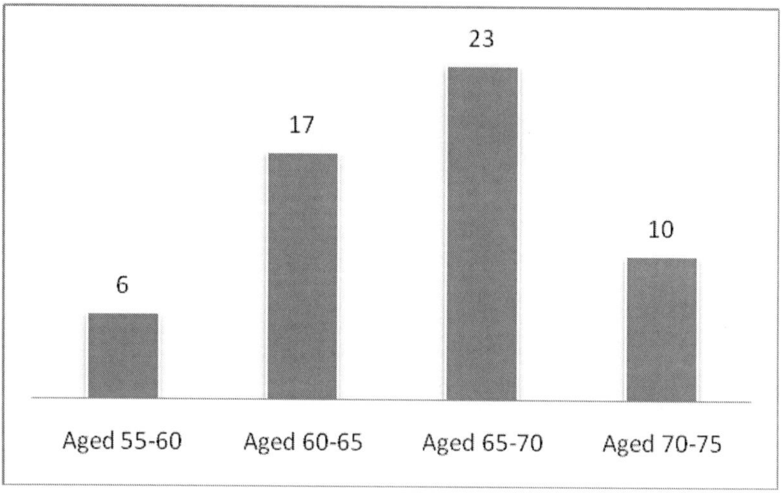

Figure 2-1. Number of participants per age range

Figure 2-2 below shows the number of British retirees surveyed by length of stay. The groups are very homogeneous in terms of the number of participants in each.

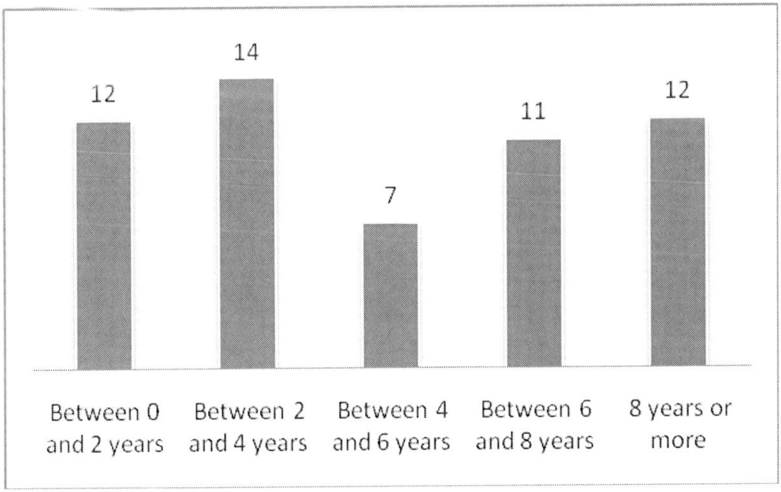

Figure 2-2. Number of British retirees surveyed by length of stay

Figure 2-3 below displays the mean of LLS per category used by the participants of the study. Social strategies predominate among the other categories with 3.9 out of 5.

Figure 2-4 below shows how the length of the stay can be a factor for the overall use of strategies. There is a tendency for the LLS use to increase with time spent in the country, ending with 4.1 out of 5 for those participants with 8 or more years in the country of destination.

Conclusions and Suggestions

Living abroad seems to be a challenging activity, especially when the local language represents an issue. Experience plays an important role, and the longer a foreign retiree spends in the destination country the more LLS they use to deal with the inconvenience of the lack of knowledge of the local language. The "social strategies" seem to have special importance where the learner tries to involve native speakers of the language in their learning. The elevated use of these social strategies indicates a strong will to integrate and network. Although age does not appear to consistently change the use of any LLS category, it is true that the older the participant the less use they make of strategies which *a posteriori* could be an indicator of lack of interest in learning the local language or integrating. Retirees over a certain age might think that it is too late or that it is too much effort to learn another language, especially if they are old enough to consider that they are not going to enjoy this commodity for a long time.

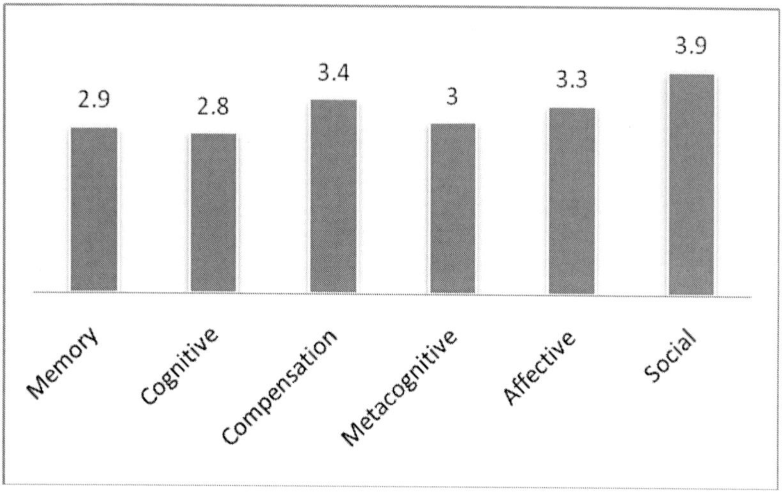

Figure 2-3. Mean of LLS per category used by the participants of the study

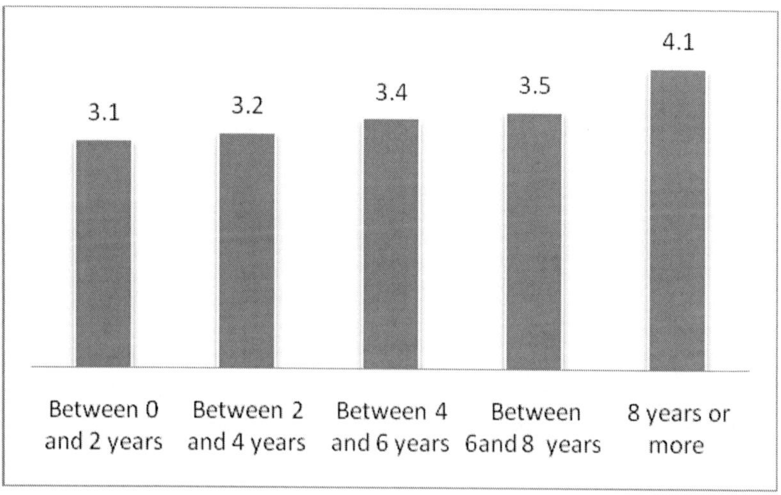

Figure 2-4. Length of the stay can be a factor for the overall use of strategies

Future lines of research can contemplate the possibility of looking closer into the interpersonal skills of the participants. In other words, they can construct the concepts of introversion and extroversion in people and apply it to the use of LLS and their different categories. Furthermore, other factors such as socioeconomic status or previous academic or professional experiences abroad can be observed for a similar impact of the use of LLS. Finally, the execution of this study observed that some elderly people do not worry about networking or connecting with locals, mainly because of the big number of individuals and families of the same nationality or social clubs.

References

Anthias, F. (2006). Belonging in a Globilising and Unequal World: Rethinking Translocations. In N. Yuvaldavis, K. Kannabiran & U. Vieten, *The Situated Politics of Belonging*. London: Sage.

Betty, C. & Cahill, M. (1997). Language problems of older British migrants on the Costa del Sol. *Generations Review 7 (2):* 10-11.

Birdsong, D. (Ed.). (1999). *Second language acquisition and the critical period hypothesis*. London: Psychology Press.

Bornstein, M. H. (1989). Sensitive periods in development: Structural characteristics and causal interpretations. *Psychological Bulletin 105*: 179-197.

Casado-Díaz, M. A., Kaiser, C. & Warnes, A. M. (2004). Northern European retired residents in nine southern European areas: characteristics, motivations and adjustment. *Ageing and Society 24 (3)*: 353-381.

Cuba, L. & Longino, C. (1991). Regional retirement migration: the case of Cape Cod. *Journal of Gerontology 46 (1)*: 533-542.

Friedrich, K. & Warnes, A. (2000). Understanding contacts in later life migration patterns: Germany, Britain and the United States. *Erdkunde 54:* 108-120.

Glasgow, N. (1995). Retirement migration and the use of services in non-metropolitan counties. *Rural Sociology 60 (2)*: 224-243.

—. Hardill, IPLEASE INSERT AUTHORS NAME. *Online government—Offline older people: Prof Irene Hardill presentation.* Online: http://www,cardi.ie/publications/onlinegovernmentofflineolderpeopleprofirenehardillpresentation.

King, R., Warnes, A. & Williams, A. (1998).International retirement migration in Europe. *International Journal of Population Geography 4 (2)*: 97-111.

Newport, E. (1991). Contrasting conceptions of the critical period for language. In S. Carey & R. Gelman (Eds.), The epigenesist of mind: Essays on biology and cognition. Hillsdale, NJ: Lawrence Erlbaum Associates. 111-130.

Rowles, G. & Watkins, J. (1993). Elderly migration and development in small communities. *Growth and Change 24 (3)*: 509-538.

MINORITIES' ISSUES IN RELATION TO THE RIGHT TO SELF-DETERMINATION

CLAUDIA-LIVIA ANDRIŢOI

Introduction

The minorities issue is extremely complex, being specific to the contemporary world. Minorities have always existed, but along with the emergence of democracy as a universal value towards the end of the eighteenth century, minorities became a serious political and social problem, also playing a major part in international relations. Thus, the modern variant of humanitarianism and law tried to temper the sharpening of minority conflicts, offering protection, by international treaties, to ethnic, linguistic or religious minorities. The term of minority—more precisely a linguistic, ethnic, religious minority—designates the human groups in a position of numerical inferiority, without exception, and at the same time in political, social, economic or cultural inferiority. The fact of being a minority also implies being minor from the legal or sociologic viewpoint. In other words, it is necessary to take into consideration a quantitative and differentiating reality, as well as a condition of a real dependence or a dependency felt as such.

Methods and Techniques

The research methods used in this study have an important role in the identification of the scientific ground underlying the theories elaborated in this field. Furthermore, they aim at clarifying the concepts approached, which are extremely important in grasping the essence of law. The epistemological method plays an essential part in identifying the particularities at the basis of the norms of law maintained until now on the legal plane, insisting on the degree of precision conferred to scientific research, and thus justifying the use of the legal methodology as a set of norms of selection, co-operation and appreciation of advantages and, possibly, of the drawbacks of applying each of these methods. Other research methods used are: the interpretative method, the structuralist-systematic method necessary for the awareness of the organisation and functioning of law as a system of social organisation orienting scientific knowledge, and the operations, procedures and techniques of this knowledge. Legal logic is a component of the legal methodology and interpretation, being a precise subject, through its regulation object, and its useful results. By legal or juridical logic we understand the theory of sources or the idea of source of law. It comprises mythology or the ideas, legal sociology or the data, and nomology or the constructs.

Present Concerns for the Protection of Minorities

The idea underlying this survey is along three dimensions:

- Construction, over a long time, of historic minorities—a dimension constituting time/duration or genesis. The origin of minorities becomes an important factor for their differentiation.
- The second dimension would be the impact of minorities on space through the constitution and preservation, during shorter or longer periods, of minority territories or regionalisms. This impacts the internal policy of states in terms of diversity, evoking complexity, regionalisation, internal autonomy, provincial regimes and federalism, experiences engaging the state in the relation with minorities. Federalism as internal institutional variable, regional policy decentralisation, and acknowledgement of linguistic cultural or religious particulars may lead however to the reality of unequal economic development, to the disparity of social conditions—variables intervening in the constitution of the state's policies regarding minorities.
- A third dimension consists in the dynamics of movement creating new minorities, such as exodus, professional migration, etc.

Each of these aspects implies taking into account, simultaneously, the minorities' aspirations and claims, as well as their attitudes to the majority surrounding society, in the legal sense of the term.

The purpose of this chapter joins the search for answers to the question: "What does it mean to examine the dispositions to adopt for defining the principles applicable in the field of fight against minorities' discrimination and minorities' protection?" The answer is nuanced, because when the commission for human rights decided on the establishment of a single sub-commission for the prevention of minority discrimination and their protection, its mandate was also set, but in general terms it established the examination of dispositions to be adopted for defining the applied principles in the domain of the fight against discriminating measures based on race, gender, language or religion, and in the domain of minorities' protection, together with forwarding recommendations to the Commission about the urgent issues in these fields (Mihăilă 2006, 125).

The existence and reanimation of national, linguistic or religious minorities—ethnic-cultural minorities—open the debate, in various degrees, about the political and social equilibriums in multiple sectors of the contemporary world. Laponce distinguishes between minorities that are ready to accept their status (of minority) from the desire to preserve identity—minorities by will—and minorities that seek insurance against assimilation by the dominant groups—minorities by force. Wirth makes the distinction among minorities which are assimilationist (willing to be assimilated), pluralist (desire to remain distinct), secessionist (desire for separation) and militant (wish to turn the dominant group into a minority) (Sudre 2006, 89). The enumeration of typologies can continue—what is essential is that, compared to dominant groups, minorities differ according to their relative size, their distinct features (national, ethnic religious or linguistic), their purposes (acculturation, integration or separation), and according to obstacles, if any, that the dominant group raises in reaching these goals (Diaconu 1996, 78).

A particular case of minorities is represented by national minorities. According to contemporary researches, they are the result of incorporation into a new, larger state of a previous self-governance (Kymlicka), majorities becoming political minorities as a result of the state frontier remodelling. National minorities are characterised by the desire to preserve themselves as distinct societies. Roger Brubaker forwards interesting details, defining minorities as dynamic political attitudes or families of mutual attitudes in competition. Three elements are characteristic for the family of attitudes:

- Public support of belonging to an ethnic-cultural nation distinct from the nation that is numerically or politically dominant
- Claims directed at the state to recognise the ethnic-cultural distinction of the nationality
- On the basis of ethic-cultural nationality, the demand of collective cultural and/or political rights.

The issue of minorities' rights reached the core position it occupies today within international relations only after the end of First World War. The fluidity of inter-community conflicts in Central Europe, culminating with the assassination, in 1914, of Archduke Ferdinand of Austria, at Sarajevo, is generally considered the spark that triggered the explosion of the "Great War." The desire to attenuate that conflict and impose the observance of the frontiers retraced after the war led to the establishment of minorities' regimes. It was a system initially imposed on the defeated by the winning powers, uninterested in a general regime of minority protection, i.e. one that would apply restrictions in the way the triumphant powers treated their own minorities themselves.

The present interest in minority protection comes from the approach of the problem after the Second World War in Eastern Europe. After a period of a massive transfer of population, in which the Allies were involved or to which they consented, the minorities' movements were effectively suppressed. Despite the existence of constitutional structures of a federal nature (like Yugoslavia or the Soviet Union), that could even contemplate to right to secession, the reality of totalitarian leadership, by a single party, impeded most social differences to find their political expression. The minorities' aspirations were especially frozen. However, the ice covering them during the Cold War did not destroy them. On the contrary, they were perfectly conserved on an unfulfilled agenda. Along with the renouncing to the Soviet control in Eastern Europe and the collapse of the Soviet Union itself, together with the end of the Cold War, the possibility was opened of returning to older priorities.

Guiding Principles in the Protection of Minorities

In the present stage of international law evolution, three great principles were imposed to the international community regarding issues related to minorities and human rights.

The first recognised general principle is that each state is sovereign on its territory or that the human rights issues are of its competence and must be solved without foreign interference, by the authorities of the respective state.

The second principle is that the citizens belonging to national minorities must not be persecuted or discriminated against; they must benefit from rights equal to those of their own citizens and also ensure the preservation of the cultural identity, see their traditions and lifestyles respected, with any attempt to annihilate their rights or to "assimilate" them into the majority population being inadmissible.

The third principle is that of international co-operation of states in the domain of minorities' rights, postulating the firm adhesion of all countries to a set of generally recognised principles, corresponding to a certain international standard, excluding the autarchic or exclusionist positions, and of "rejection" of any preoccupations from the part of the international community in relation to the minorities' situation.

This is the approach brought about by the intentional law of human rights, although, in general, it protects the socio-economic rights less and the civil and political rights more. The key stipulation is art. 27 of the Pact regarding civil and political rights: "in the states where there are ethnic, religious or linguistic minorities, the persons belonging to these minorities cannot be deprived of the right to have, in common with the other members of their group, their own cultural life, to practice their own religion or to use their own language."

Furthermore, the declaration regarding the rights of persons belonging to national, ethic, religious and linguistic minorities also refers to such persons as having: "the right to enjoy their own culture, to profess and practice their own religion and to use their own language." This wording can be comprehended as a strengthening of the article 27 approach. The covered spheres of activity raise a special interest regarding culture, religion and language. It is a short list, but it grasps the essence of what seems to be the defining characteristic of the minorities involved in the types of conduct, having provoked a major political preoccupation.

At this point, the problem can be restricted to a declaration made of one of the pact signatory states. At the moment of the Pact ratification, France declared that "in the light of art. 2 of the French Republic Constitution, art. 27 cannot be applied as regards the French Republic." The aforementioned constitutional stipulation states that France "is an indivisible, secular, democratic and social republic. It will ensure the equality of all citizens before the law, without distinction of origin, race or religion. It will respect all convictions." By invoking this principle, France claimed that it had "no minorities."

The idea seems to be that acknowledging the existence of minorities, in order to correspond to the goals set by art. 27 of the Pact, is incompatible with the text of art. 2 of the French Constitution. That principle, in one form or another, is present not only in the French legal system, but also in many national constitutions, and in several of the pact stipulations. Nevertheless, only France formulated such a declaration. An explanation offered by an authorised commentator, Alfred de Zayas, is that France did not want "to assume any obligations to affirmative action, i.e. to ensure legal equality and in fact, by adequate positive measures."

The question appears of what "possible measures" can be required, and if these measures would be required by the provisions of the pact anyway, including referring to the non-discrimination and equal treatment before the law.

There are two such provisions. The first is article 2: "The signatory states of this Pact commit themselves to respect and guarantee all individuals on their territory and who are of their competence, the rights recognised in the present Pact, without discrimination, especially of race, colour, gender, language, political opinion or any other opinion, national or social origin, wealth, birth, or based on any other circumstances." The difficulty in this situation is the reaffirmation of the already existing human rights. They do not constitute a law *per se*. Its counterpart in the European Convention of Human Rights is art. 14.

Comparatively, art. 26 of the Pact stipulates that: "All persons are equal before the law and have, without discrimination, the right to equal protection of the law. Thus, the law must forbid any discrimination and guarantee all persons equal and effective protection against any discrimination, namely race, colour, gender, language, religion, political opinion or any other opinion, national or social origin, wealth, birth or founded on any other circumstances." This is a self-standing article, independent of any other provisions, stipulating the autonomous right to equality before the law and non-discriminations. It has no counterpart in the European Convention. The UN organism in charge of the minorities' protection is the sub-commission for the prevention of discrimination and protection of minorities.

This is one of the four sub-commissions intended for creation by the Economic and Social Council since the beginning of its activity, i.e. the sub-commissions: for women's conditions, for freedom of information and press, for protection of minorities and for prevention of discrimination. When the problem rose to effectively constituting the sub-commission for the women's conditions, the Economic and Social Council conferred it the status of commission, and by Resolution no. 9 (II) of July 21, 1946, the council conferred the right of the commission for human rights to establish a sub-commission for the freedom of information and press, a sub-commission for the protection of minorities, and a sub-commission for the prevention of discrimination.

The commission for human rights decided, during its first reunion of January to February 1947, to create only two sub-commissions instead of three, i.e. the sub-commission for the prevention of discrimination and protection of minorities, and the sub-commission for the freedom of information and press. The sub-commission for the prevention of discrimination and protection of minorities is made of independent experts, who function on their own behalf. They are proposed by the sates and selected by the commission, after consultations with the secretary general, for a three-year period— the governments control the competence of the sub-commission through the Commission for Human Rights. As remarked in the literature, no mandatory definitional character was given, by treaties or by any main UN organism, to the notions of "prevention of discrimination and protection of minorities," apart from what the sub-commission stated in relation to these notions. It was highlighted thus that "the prevention of discrimination consists in preventing any actions denying individuals or groups of persons the equality of treatment they should enjoy," whereas the protection of minorities means "the protection of groups that are not dominant in a state who, aiming at being treated in conditions of equality, generally, with the majority, wish, to a certain extent, a distinct treatment, ensuring them the preservation of the fundamental features differentiating them from the majority population." It is also pointed out that such characteristics are based on race, religion and language.

The UN Secretary General drew up a memorandum accepted by the sub-commission, in which he defined the relations between the two activities of preventing discrimination and protecting minorities. If, theoretically, the problems contained in this document are logical, in practice they do not lead to the best results, keeping in mind the numerous political or other types of considerations impeding their application (the fact that minorities usually claim both equality and differentiated treatment at the same time, or the reluctance of some governments to accept minorities and their specific rights). As regards the prevention of discrimination, the sub-commission had the task of analysing the draft of articles related to non-discrimination, established by the commission to be included in the Universal Declaration of Human Rights, and in this sense it proposed the addition of further criteria underlying the identification of discrimination of political opinions or opinions of other natures, material conditions, and social or national origin.

Moreover, the sub-commission dealt with the discrimination issue as regards the right to emigration and free movement of persons, stipulated in art. 13 of the Universal Declaration of Human Rights, the respective studies being especially oriented against the socialist and some third-world countries. The increase in the number of third-world countries in the UN and its organisms determined a change in the vote results related to different problems regarding the prevention of discrimination, and some attempts by certain states to prevent the adoption of certain measures failed. The Sub-Commission proceeded to the appointment of special reporting experts for the issues constituting the object of its studies (Năstase 1998, 35).

The other dimension of the sub-commission mandate refers to the protection of minorities. As from the drafts of the Universal Declaration of Human Rights, those stipulations referring to certain rights granted to minorities were removed, so that the declaration no longer contains any referral in this respect, and the sub-commission's attention was also drawn to that direction. In fact, the UN General Assembly adopted, as a compromise solution, a resolution summoning the Sub-Commission "to draw up a study on the issue of minorities so that the UN could take effective measures for the protection of racial, national, religious or linguistic minorities." We should, however, remark that this resolution was elaborated to calm the situation, because in reality, for a long period, neither the General Assembly nor other UN organisms manifested any especial interest for the adoption of international regulations and for taking efficient measures for minorities' protection, a situation caused by the different political considerations and the states' contradictory interests.

Under these circumstances, the sub-commission initiated studies regarding the definition of minorities and their classification according to the protection they need, and obtained information related to the situation of minorities in the UN member states. Attempting to replace the absence from the Universal Declaration of Human Rights of a disposition regarding minorities, the sub-commission acted for the introduction into the pact regarding political and civil rights of art. 27, which confers minorities the right to culture, religion and language.

After the adoption of the pact, the sub-commission appointed a special reporting expert to draw up a study related to the implications of art. 27 on the international plane. This report, when completed, contained a series of observations and conclusions related to the modality in which states have to apply these dispositions, and the obstacles encountered (Bârsan 2005, 34). Considering that the commission intended to elaborate a declaration draft regarding minorities, it asked the sub-commission, in 1984, to prepare a definition of "minority." In 1985 an analysis in this sense was presented, but its debate was contradictory regarding many of its aspects and elements, and is reason why it was not accepted. The activity carried on by the UN through its organisms specialised in this domain were concretised by the adoption of the declaration regarding the rights of persons who belong to national, ethnic, religious or linguistic minorities.

As for the European continent, the member states of the Council of Europe, considering that the turmoil of the European history had shown that the protection of national minorities is essential for the stability, democratic security and peace of the continent, they adopted on February 1, 1995 the convention-frame for the protection of national minorities. From the convention's perspective, the protection of national minorities and rights and liberties of the persons belonging to these minorities are an intrinsic part of the international protection of human rights, thus constituting a domain of international co-operation.

On the grounds of this document, the parties pledge themselves to adopt, if need be, adequate measures to promote, in all domains of economic, social, political and cultural life, full and effective equality between the persons belonging to a national minority and the persons belonging to the majority. Furthermore, they will encourage the spirit of tolerance and intercultural dialogue and will take effective measures for promoting mutual respect, understanding and co-operation among all the persons living on their territory, irrespective of the ethnic, cultural, linguistic or religious identities, especially in the domain of education, culture and information media. Each person belonging to a national minority will be recognised regarding the right to freely use, without interference, their minority languages, in private and in public, orally and in writing. They will have equal opportunities of access to education on all levels, to cultural, social and economic life and to public affairs. In turn, the persons belonging to national minorities will respect, in exercising these rights and liberties, the national legislation and the rights of the others, especially of the persons belonging to the majority or other national minorities.

The convention nevertheless points out that if the rights and liberties resulting from the principles inscribed in it are the object of a corresponding provision in the convention for the defence of human rights and fundamental rights or their afferent additional protocol, they will be understood in accordance with the latter.

Conclusions

To comprehend the phenomena related to the occurrence and evolution of the concept of human rights, we must regard this development through the prism of the events occurring along the historical stages of humankind. For this historic incursion, we need to resort to the evolution of philosophic thinking, knowledge process and aptitudes characteristic to humans, who are endowed with reason. The level of human rights protection reached today is the fruit of a long history that traversed several stages from time immemorial. Starting with the idea that the individual fundamental rights are consecrated either in the constitutions of different countries or by international documents which, grace to the prestige acquired, were imposed to the general respect, the Aix Colloquy of January 1981 considered that, by the notion of fundamental individual rights, we must understand "the set of rights and liberties recognised both to natural persons and to legal persons (of private and public law) in virtue of the Constitution and international texts, and protected both against the executive power and against the legislative power by the constitutional judge (or the international judge)." The distinction between human rights exercised individually and those exercised in common with others starts from the assertion that what characterises certain rights is the fact they cannot be exercised by the isolated action of one person, but necessarily suppose the participation of certain manifestations of concordant will from the part of other subjects enjoying the same rights. If we take into consideration this uncontested reality, we will have to reach the conclusion that when a series of international documents speak about the right of peoples to dispose of themselves, to establish their own political status, to dispose freely of their natural riches and resources, etc., they start from the very idea of the existence of the category of individual rights exercised in common, by a community.

References

Bârsan, C. (2005). *Convenţia europeană a drepturilor omului I* [European Convention of human rights 1]. Bucureşti: All Beck.

Diaconu, I. (1996). *Minorităţile—statut şi perspective* [Minorities: status and perspectives]. Bucureşti: IRDO.

Mihăilă, M. (2006). *Tratat de drept internaţional public III* [Treaty of international public law III]. Bucureşti: BREN—V.I.S.PRINT.

Năstase, A. (1998). *Drepturile persoanelor aparţinând minorităţilor naţionale* [Rights of persons belonging to national minoritie]. Bucureşti: Official Gazette.

Sudre, F. (2006). *Drept european şi internaţional al drepturilor omului* [European and international law of human rights]. Iaşi: Polirom.

THE RIGHT TO SELF-DETERMINATION IN THE INTERNATIONAL AREA

MARIAN MIHĂILĂ

Introduction

All peoples have the right to determine, in full freedom, their internal and external political status, without intervention from abroad, and to achieve, according to their own free will, their political, economic, social and cultural development, on the condition they observe the territorial integrity and preserve the existing frontiers.

These new categories of human rights determine the international organisms to approach them within certain legal instruments, given the continuous evolution of human society, the complexity of issues they have to face, and especially as a reaction to some generalised perils.

In virtue of this principle, peoples have the right to constitute themselves in a national state, to freely choose and develop their political, economic and social system, without outside interference, and have the right to permanent sovereignty over their natural resources. Moreover, the right to self-determination is also encountered under other formulations, such as: "peoples' rights to dispose of themselves," "peoples' equality in rights" and "peoples' right to dispose of themselves." Irrespective of denomination, this right is recognised, on the international plane, as one of the fundamental human rights.

Research Methods

The research methods used in the study were: the historic method, the conceptualist method, the logic method and the intuitive method, necessary as reasoning means in view of arguing the demonstration. Other research methods were the conceptualist method, the logic method and the intuitive method necessary as means of reasoning for argument purposes. The research methods and techniques are systematically presented on the model of argumentation *in utramque partem*, i.e. of contrary principles, which oppose each other, although a couple are developed that cannot be dissociated; on the contrary, the components extract their significance from the dualist structure where they belong, as we shall argue in the study below (Andrițoi 2010, 105).

The Self-Determination Principle

The apparition and evolution of the self-determination concept can be traced back to the period of multi-national empires, i.e. the nineteenth century. The principle of self-determination occurs as the successor of the political principle of nationality which, in the eighteenth and nineteenth centuries, turned the ethnic and linguistic identity into the basis of political unity. The liberal authors considered the self-government liberty of national communities as a premise necessary for individual freedoms as, in their opinion, there is an intrinsic connection between the individual's liberty and their belonging to a national community. The national state was considered the adequate and necessary frame for the guarantee of the rights of citizens living in multi-national empires. As sovereignty is also expressed in the peoples' right to self-determination, nations were entitled to claim this right (Sudre 2006, 89).

Public opinion held that self-determination was related to independence. It is believed that in the United Nations Charter, self-determination is treated as a decisive step toward independence. However, this does not correspond to the truth. First, when the United Nations Charter was adopted there were fifty-one members, all independent. Second, the reason for the approach of peoples that were not yet independent was related to the acknowledgement of the fact that colonial powers had duties toward the governed peoples. Consequently, the issue of granting independence to former colonies was considered a very thorny problem. We shall examine different stages of the self-determination process:

- The first stage—self-determination and independence from under the colonial domination. Other documents about the economic and social co-operation of the United Nations pledged themselves to ensure the universal respect of human rights with the purpose of creating the necessary conditions for peaceful and friendly relations among nations "based on equality in rights and self-determination." The context where these articles are placed is important. Both in article 1 (2) and in other articles, we read about the rights of peoples in a state to be protected from the interference of another state or government. The self-determination concept did not refer to the right of independence of dependant peoples. It is obvious that the evolution of the self-determination concept is historically related to decolonisation and the increasingly general agreement on the obligation to ensure independence for dependant peoples, if they opt for it. Although self-determination started to be accepted as a legal right in the decolonisation context, it was never restricted to the option for independence. The options of the people in one territory to unite with another state, or to remain in constitutional relations with the former colonial power, were equally accepted. The option was usually in favour of independence. The United Nations have often played an active part in the exercise of this option through the fact that they organised a referendum or a plebiscite themselves, or by the monitoring of their exercise (Diaconu 1996, 78).

- The second phase—self-determination beyond colonialism and human rights. The following phase in the legal evolution was the establishment of a convention between self-determination as a legal obligation in the decolonisation process and self-determination as a human right. Two resolutions of the General Assembly, adopted at an interval of twenty-four hours from one another, speak about the rights of people to self-determination. Resolution 1514 (XV) of the General Assembly, and the Resolution 1541 (XV) of the General Assembly. Resolution 1541 (XV) clarified that this exercise of self-determination can result in different solutions, and stipulated that the process required guarantees that the option would be free, voluntary and in full awareness. However, six years after the adoption of this key resolution about decolonisation, the rights to self-determination came to be seen as a self-standing precept, exceeding the limit of normative practices from the decolonisation domain.

As regards the two international pacts related to the economic, social and cultural rights, and to the civil and political rights respectively, concluded in 1966, as well as other international, universal and regional documents, they consecrated the right of peoples as a norm of international law regarding friendly relations and co-operation among states.

Formulated identically, article I in the two pacts reads:

- All the peoples have the right to dispose of themselves, in virtue of this right they freely determine their political status and freely ensure their economic, social and cultural development.
- In order to reach their goals, all the peoples can freely dispose of their natural riches and resources, without prejudicing the

obligations resulted from the international economic co-operation, based on the principles of mutual interest and on the international law, in no circumstance a people cannot be deprived of their own living means.

- The signatory states of the present Pact, including those which have the responsibility of the administration of non-autonomous territories and territories under tutorship, must facilitate the realisation of peoples' right to dispose of themselves and to observe this right in accordance with the dispositions of the United Nations Chart.

The international public law thus consecrated the right of peoples to dispose of themselves as a human right.

Starting from that moment, we note the repeated referrals to self-determination in terms of human rights. The Helsinki Final Act was built on the old language of the UN Charter, clarifying at the same time that self-determination is a right of peoples. It speaks about the "principle of equal rights and self-determination of peoples," based on which "all peoples have always the right to decide, in full freedom, when and how they want, their political internal and external status, without interference from abroad, and to follow, in accordance with their free will, their own political, economic, social and cultural development." Although self-determination has evolved, since its modest beginning in the United National Charter, from a legal entitlement to decolonisation to a self-standing human right, there are many questions that still need to find answers (Bârsan 2005, 34).

The evolution of the self-determination principle led to the acknowledgement that the right to self-determination was applicable not only to the peoples under colonial domination, but to all peoples subjected to a foreign domination. This was expressed in 1970 by the Declaration of the United Nations regarding Friendship Relations. Often invoked in connection with this subject—although the declaration is rather a resolution of the General Assembly than an instrument with mandatory character and, although the two Pacts do not mention this circumstance—the declaration speaks about self-determination as being a possibility in the situations of colonialism and for "the peoples subjected to foreign subjugation, domination or exploitation." Those who supported this clause clearly had two distinct circumstances in mind. The first regarded South Africa, an independent state, but considered by many as being subjected to "foreign domination," and having foreign support for the domination over the minority. The second was a matter of a totally different nature—the status of occupied territories after the end or suspension of military operations. The need was felt that the position of peoples in these territories be protected not only through humanitarian law, but also through the insistence on their right to self-determination. In any case, there were many United Nations resolutions referring to the right to self-determination in the circumstances of foreign occupation.

For a considerable period of time there was a serious resistance to the suggestion that self-determination could apply in any way outside the colonial context. This reluctance was shared by Eastern European states and the new territories. The phenomenon was acceptable only in the case of decolonisation, and many of the new states considered self-determination as a problem between them and their former colonial masters, and not one between them and their own population.

Partially, the third-world states feared that post-colonial self-determination would necessarily result in the fragmenting of the new national states, the ethnic groups from a state resorting to secession attempts and eventually uniting with the same ethnic population from another country. However, the idea that self-determination has a general applicability was massively supported by the Committee for Human Rights, acting according to the Pact on Civil and Political Rights, and this idea has, without doubt, exercised a general influence.

Considering that "the rights of peoples and nations to dispose of themselves is a prior condition for them to enjoy all fundamental human rights," the UN General Assembly made the member states the following recommendations in 1952:

- To support this principle
- To recognise and favour the achievement of human rights for the persons inhabiting the non-autonomous territories and the territories under tutorship under their authority to dispose of themselves and of the exercise of this right
- To take practical measures to prepare the respective peoples in view of exercising this right and to ensure the participation of autochthonous populations in the legislative and executive organisms of the respective territory
- To supply information on the measures taken in view of leading these territories, in the shortest delay possible, to the stage of autonomy or independence.

An important moment was the year 1960, when this principle, the right to self-determination, was more and more promoted and reaffirmed, evolution which culminated on December 14 in the moment when the General Assembly adopted the "Declaration regarding the granting of independence to colonial countries and peoples" by Resolution no. 1514, proclaiming "the necessity to put an end, immediately and unconditionally, to colonialism under all its forms and manifestations," as well as the obligation of states to immediately grant independence to the countries and peoples from colonies. The year 1960 was the year when twelve former colonies acquired independence and joined the free states' community (Andriţoi 2010, 125).

The Trichotomic Structure of the Self-Determination Right

The self-determination right is one of the fundamental principles of international law and defined in art. 1 of the UN charter, the pillar of international law after the Second World War, as having two dimensions:

- The internal aspect of self-determination, more precisely the right of peoples to freely determine their political status and to develop from the economic, social and cultural viewpoint
- The external aspect of acknowledging the right of peoples to determine their place in the international community of states and the relations with them.

Concretely, all the above means that peoples have the right to constitute a state, and the latter establishes its external co-operation as it chooses. Whenever a state appears on the world map, we can say about the international community that it recognised the existence of a new people enjoying the exercise or the right to self-determination. Vice versa, whenever the international community recognises a group of people as being "a people," it also accepts that this group of persons has the right to found a state. The fact that in the logic of international law we have a biunivocal relation between "people" and "state" represents the key for understanding the political-identity problems in today's world (Năstase 1998, 35). From the charter, as well as, for instance, from the French Declaration of Rights of 1795, reading that "Each people is independent and sovereign, irrespective of the number of individuals that compose it and the size of the territory they occupy," we cannot find too much about the meaning of "people." However, we can understand from art. 1 of the charter that it is about entities exercising sovereign rights, as only the states are subjects of international law, bearers of rights and obligations. The text does not leave room for another interpretation: "The purposes of the United Nations are to develop friendly relations among nations, based on the respect for the principle of equal rights and self-determination of peoples." Art. 1 of the International Pact regarding the Civil and Political Rights means that we can speak about entities which exercise certain forms of authority. The same article also contains a reference to the non-autonomous territories and territories under tutorship as beneficiaries of the rights stipulated in the charter. It is clear that the International Pact regarding the Civil and Political Rights falls within the same range of stipulations strengthened by the UN charter. However, we have not yet defined the criteria according to which we could find out which peoples, beside those previously mentioned, could claim the right to self-determination stipulated in the texts of the charter and the pact (Andriţoi 2010, 155). One of the details that interest us can be found in general comment no. 23 of the International Pact regarding civil and political rights, adopted in New York on April 6, 1994 by the UN Committee for Human Rights, with the purpose of eliminating the confusions provoked by the application of art. 27 in the pact referring to the rights of persons belonging to ethnic, religious or linguistic minorities. Point two of the comment states the following: "in some communications subjected to the attention of the Committee, based on the facultative Protocol, the right recognised in art. 27 was confused with the right of peoples to self-determination proclaimed by art. 1 of the Pact." For this reason, point 3.1. of the comment establishes that:

> The Pact provides a distinction between the right to self-determination and the rights protected by art. 27. The former appears as a right belonging to peoples and is treated in a separate section of the Pact (Part I). Self-determination is not a right that can be capitalised within the additional Protocol. On the other hand, art. 27 refers to rights belonging to individuals as such and is included, like the articles referring to other personal rights conferred to individuals in Part III of the Pact that can be capitalised based on the stipulations of the additional Protocol.

The clarification brought about by the adoption of the general comment is valuable in the fact that it establishes the distinction between peoples and national minorities, but it is partial and does not help to define the elements underlying the concept of "people" used in the charter and pact texts. The document providing the most information is the Draft of the Declaration regarding the rights of native peoples, finalised in 1994 by the UN Sub-Commission for the prevention of discrimination and protection of minorities. Paragraph 1, Part I of the Declaration Draft consecrates the right of native peoples to self-determination, in accordance with the international law and based on the status and political institutions they can freely establish and their economic, social and cultural development they can freely choose. An intrinsic part of this right is the right to autonomy and self-government. Paragraph 3, Part I of the Declaration Draft sets the right of native peoples to be free and equal with other human communities or peoples in dignity and rights.

Conclusions

From the analysis of the previous texts it follows that the documents adopted until 1965 recognised the right to self-determination only for the peoples from the non-autonomous territories and the territories under tutorship. By the two international pacts of 1966 this right is recognised to all peoples. The right to self-determination thus belongs to all peoples, both those who live in countries that have not yet acquired independence and within states, instituting one of the elements of the democratic institutions that must function in virtue of the will freely expressed by all citizens of the respective state. The content of the right to self-determination is tripled to political, economic and human. As regards the political content, it is expressed by several elements:

- it is about, first of all, the right of peoples that are subjected to any form of domination or dependency to constitute their own state. For this purpose, they can resort to any means, peaceful or violent. The armed conflicts in which peoples fight against the colonial domination, foreign occupation and the racist regimes are conflicts with international characters and are governed by the international humanitarian law.
- observance of the territorial integrity and preservation of existing frontiers.

The economic content refers to the permanent sovereignty of peoples over their natural riches and resources. It was stated as a principle of international law in a series of legal and diplomatic documents related to the fundamental human rights. After the UN General Assembly created the Commission for the permanent sovereignty over their natural resources in 1958, on December 14, 1962 it adopted Resolution no. 1803 which contains a series of rules referring to the mode of exercising the respective right as a fundamental element of the right of peoples to dispose of themselves, among which:

- the right to permanent sovereignty of peoples and nations over their natural riches and reserves must be exercised in the interest of the national development and wellbeing of the interested state
- the prospecting, capitalising and disposing of these resources, and the importance of foreign capitals necessary for this purpose, must be in accordance with the rules and conditions in which the peoples and nations consider, in full freedom, as being necessary or recommendable in relation with the authorisation, limitations or interdiction of these activities
- nationalisation, expropriation or requisition will have to be founded on reasons or motives of public utility, security or national interest, recognised as having priority over the mere individual or private interests, both national and foreign
- the international co-operation in view of developing the economy of developing countries must favour the independent national development of these countries and be grounded on the observance of their sovereignty
- the violation of the sovereign rights of peoples and nations over their natural riches and resources is contrary to the spirit and principles of the UN Charter and hinders the development of international co-operation and preservation of peace.

The United Nations Conference on the Environment and the UN Conference on commerce and development adopted, in 1972, decisions regarding the permanent sovereignty over natural resources. The Stockholm Conference on the environment announced, in the adopted declaration, the principles that the states have the sovereign right to exploit their own resources according to their environment policy and have the duty to act so that the activities exercised within the limit of their jurisdiction or under their control should not harm the environment of other states or regions that do not belong to any national jurisdiction. The UN Conference on commerce and development (UNCTAD) adopted the Charter of Economic Rights and Duties of States, which especially affirms the right to permanent sovereignty of states over their natural resources. After 1974, when the problem of "the permanent sovereignty over natural resources in the Arab occupied territories" was indicated to the UN General Assembly, the Resolution adopted in 1977 underlined the right of Arab states whose territories were under Israeli occupation to exercise their sovereignty and control in a complete, effective and permanent manner all their natural resources and of other nature, their riches and economic activities. The assembly reaffirmed that all the measures taken by Israel to exploit the resources from the Arab occupied territories were illegal, and also the right of Arab states and peoples to be returned their natural and human resources and all other resources, as well as the right to a full indemnity for the exploitation, exhaustion, losses and damages suffered. The principles regarding the permanent sovereignty over natural resources are also consecrated in the Charter of Economic Rights and Duties of States, which, in art. 2, affirms that: "each state owns and exercises freely its permanent and full sovereignty, including the possession, use and disposition over its entire richness, natural recourses and economic activities." Art. 3 reads: "in the exploitation of natural resources common to two or several countries, each state must co-operate based on a system of prior information and consultations, in order to ensure the optimum use of such resources, without prejudicing the legitimate interests of other states." Among other documents treating this subject we can also count "The Declaration and action program regarding the instauration of the new international economic order," adopted by the UN General Assembly at the Sixth Extraordinary Session by the resolutions 3201 (S-VI) and 3202 (S-VI) of May 1, 1974,[17] Resolution 3016/XXVII, on December 18, 1972 regarding the permanent sovereignty of developing countries over their natural resources.

References

Andriţoi, C. (2010). *Principiile interpretării în ordinea juridică pozitivă* [Principles of interpretation in the positive legal order]. Bucureşti: BREN—V.I.S.PRINT.

Bârsan, C. (2005). *Convenţia europeană a drepturilor omului I* [European Convention of human rights 1]. Bucureşti: All Beck.

Diaconu, I. (1996). *Minorităţile—statut şi perspective* [Minorities: status and perspectives]. Bucureşti: IRDO.

Năstase, A. (1998). *Drepturile persoanelor aparţinând minorităţilor naţionale* [Rights of persons belonging to national minoritie]. Bucureşti: Official Gazette.

Sudre, F. (2006). *Drept european şi internaţional al drepturilor omului* [European and international law of human rights]. Iaşi: Polirom.

NARRATIVE IDENTITIES IN BANAT, ROMANIA: THE SOCIAL REPRESENTATION OF CONFRONTATION WITH TRAUMA

ALIN GAVRELIUC AND DANA GAVRELIUC

Introduction

At the beginning of the 2000s we began a series of studies concerning the analysis of the Banatian imaginary identitary, especially for ordinary people who experienced traumatic events (like deportation), through the methodology of oral history. Years later, we have accumulated significant qualitative data around these narrative identities, and in the following we would like to briefly resume our previous attempt to outline the image of the memorial Banat (Gavreliuc 2003; 2006). The topic of traumatic identity has been followed, attempting to enlarge the horizon of the identitary knowledge toward the realm of the "silent world," and toward the "hidden" social actors like ordinary people who confront their own trauma. I am referring to approaching the simple world, which has refused the forestage of the social, a generation that has fully assumed the traumas of the last century, beginning with the great conflagrations, deportations and dramatic readjustments to post-Decembrist hopes; a generation that has accumulated so many unspoken aspirations and disillusionments and has lived each new challenge of the moment so intensely is, at last, now insisting on being listening to.

Life History and the Traumatic Self—A Qualitative Approach of Social Identities

We will resort to a privileged way of identitary journey—"the life history"—regarded as a genuine way of "producing identity live" (Kaufmann 1998, 246), in which "the confessing subject becomes a kind of concentrate of the social world," with all its hopes and failings (Elias 1991). It is proper to abandon the so-called break between the objective and subjective by understanding the social and interactive nature of the identitary construction. Consequently, they who approach this world are forced to understand that they enter a "three-pole game" (Kaufmann 1998, 240–241). It implies the researcher's empathic participation, the enjoyment and almost therapeutic unburdening of the subject, and the living and permanently rebuilt relationships with their life that become an identitary belonging for they who produce the discourse as well as for those listening to them. There is no more a place for epistemological detachment, self-sufficiency or superior considerations.

Thus, the meaning can be understood only in relation with the other who is properly considered not as a localizable and classifiable object, but as a partner in the mutual negotiation of identity as well. They become an active subject who communicates, by means of shared symbols, with another equal subject (Rostaş 1985), beside whom they get used to the "taste of the journey" among the interwoven destinies (Kaufmann 1998, 248). In this way, I will briefly outline the itinerary of such an identitary journey with a sample of interviews taken from the *Archive of the Cultural Anthropology and Oral History Group* of "The Third Europe" Foundation in Timişoara, investigated over the last decade. It offers us the opportunity to meet such a rich and ardent world by which we shall strive to catch a collective portrait of a generation that has faced so many breaks with history. Certainly, this portrait has a rather heuristic value, because of the limited samples and the inevitability of catching only one Romanian cultural area, Banat, and only one generation—adults born after 1930. We will try to clear up the tone and the essence of this journey toward the "self" and the "other" alike by examining the resources of memory.

Retrieving these fragments of life, reuniting them in a coherent ensemble, to which the subject confers referential values and significance, we will have access, by means specific to oral history, to the formation of the self as a process in this confrontation with the conditionings, often from a tragic social background and history. The life story will be looked upon as a remarkable resource of revealing the social frames of memory around which the alchemies of identity articulate. As Todorov underlined: "the representation of the past is not only the constituent part of the individual identity—the person present being, in a way, 'built' of his own self-images—but also of collective identity." Thus, "the majority of human beings need to feel they belong to a group, this being the most accessible means of obtaining the recognition of their existence, which is essential to any person" (Todorov 1998, 52–53). As American interactionism has also asserted, the narrative structure hides an argumentative structure in which the identitary discourse folds on dialogue logic. The life story assigns a part to the individual in the arena of life and also to the larger groups that have participated in the shaping of the personal destiny. Ultimately being a founding discourse, the life story constitutes a defining stage of the individual and group identity, which projects the ideology, mentality and communitarian standards and values into a new and clarifying light (Vultur & Onică 2010).

In other respects, following the manner in which the clarification of the self is achieved in this social game, Gergen introduces the term "self-narrative," by which the subject remakes their past, assembling their experience as a whole, as balanced as possible. Becoming a narrator of their own life, the subject acquires a feeling of unity and establishes a network of referential events by which the present identity appears as a dénouement of their life story (Gergen & Gergen 1988; Gergen 2009).

We do not only have a monologic formulation of discursive coherence. The identitary discourse is always addressed to the other who is listening to us. In the reading scale suggested by the symbolic interactionism, Blumer (1969) describes the way in which people act according to the significance that different social objects have for them, their significance being constructed socially within their mutual interaction and transmitted, reshaped and renewed through the process of interpretation to which social objects are submitted to and through root-images, a kind of primary constitutive elements of any semantic elaboration (interaction, the actor as a social subject and activated roles). The discovery of these deep images will constitute the main goal of the approaches I have summarised here.

This way, Bertaux reveals the valences that *le récit de vie* acquires in the knowledge of the social world or of the social situations built in the field of interactions generated by the memorial narrative. Firstly, the French anthropologist identifies the simultaneous presence of three orders of reality (Bertaux 1997): the proper socio-historical reality, with the whole ensemble of "objective" facts; the semantic reality, reuniting what the subject has acquired cognitively throughout their life, the sum of the retrospective rationalization and evaluation; and the discursive reality, which the subject formulates about their existential journey, constituting a product of a dialogue relation with one's "self" and the "other." The discursive reality takes the aspect of the story achieved depending on a series of frames (for example, the scheme of the Saviour, or of a Conspiration, supported by much more elaborated mythological structures belonging to the social imaginary). Thus, an intermediary level is interposed between the sensitive facts experienced and their telling, termed by Bertaux as the level of subjective totalization, a dynamic register, permanently made actual again, consisting of the ensemble of mental conglomerations which the subject mobilizes in order to produce a story (memories, reflections and evaluations, perspectives, and ideological elements).

Particularly, however, at the end of an oral history approach, access to the understanding of the functioning mechanism of a group's memory opens to us. This represents the clarifying instance of the definitions of realities, through which we can follow the way the transfer from individual memory to collective memory is achieved and the social identity is outlined.

Social Representation of Banatian imaginary

In the register of the final synthesis of Banatian imaginary we have used the conceptual and methodological resources of the social representation paradigm, starting with the theory of central knot and peripheral elements (Abric 1994; Flament 1989; De Rosa 2012). We have elaborated a *sui-generis* technique, combined in a matrix structure, grouping the tonality and the pregnance of the referential criteria. We have followed the exigencies required in the social representations that operate with the linguistic and conversational registers, as provided by the narrative interviews: establishing the content of representation (in our case, the image of the "Banatian identitary"), evidencing the system of categories (in our study, the identification of referential criteria) and the realising of categories (investigating the amount and the dynamics of each category).

The sampling is formed by 28 oral history interviews, including approximately 750 pages of archived manuscripts, respectively 840 printed pages. Choosing the units of analysis and carrying on the research implies the operationalization of Rokeach's social value scale (Rokeach 1973), supplemented by a content analysis. The quantitative processing has constituted only the primary stage of data interpretation. Thus, the main referential criteria of the retrospective discourse have been isolated and localized in twenty categories which in turn have been regrouped into three large thematic areas: Individual, Community/Society and Culture (see Table 2-1).

The base principle of articulating the central knot—a higher rate of frequency is the condition of its centrality—has determined us to articulate an expressive coefficient, conventionally called the "pregnance coefficient." At the same time, we have tried to take into account the specifics of our research, in which not only is the intensity of a criterion from the sample relevant, but also its orientation, evaluating through the tonality coefficient.

Table 2-1. Referential criteria resulting from content analysis

Individual	Community/society	Culture
S="self." EmV=major events in life (birth, baptism, marriage, moving house, employment, retirement, death, burial). P=personalities (a member of the family – individualized -; friend, priest, teacher, mayor). C=the "other" ethnic (German, Hungarian, Bulgarian, Gipsy); regional (Moldavian, Oltenian, Bessarabian). Ac="home." Căl=journey. D=destiny. EvTr=traumatic events (deportation, emigration, prison, exile). LR=reference places (village/town, district, street, public house). M=work.	Fam="family" (as a group or as a relation with a member of the family group). CatS=social categories (peasant, clerk, craftsman, dealer, intellectual, student, officer). SfEc=economic sphere (craftsmanship, commerce). Aut=authority (army, police, security, town hall, prefect's office). CatP=political categories (communist, iron-guardist, liberal, national-peasant, social-democrat, SS-ist). DsP=political and social discriminations (exploitation, collectivisation, class struggle).	Sb=celebrations ("rugă," "chirvai," "nedee," "fărşang"). Rel=religion (church, religious practice, faith). VCt=quotidian life (entertainment, dance, ball, fashion, sport, club, evening party, performance, film, theatre, music, choir, brass band). Ed=education ("school;" and educational code, kindergarten, school with private teachers, primary/secondary/high school, university).

We have thus developed a bi-dimensional graphic presentation which combines these two coefficients: the more consistent the pregnance is, the more the corresponding criterion will be localized closer to the origin (horizontal axis), and the more positive the tonality of the referential criterion, the closer the respective criterion will be to the same origin (vertical axis).

At the same time, if the tonality is positive, the respective referential criterion will be placed in the first dial, and if the tonality is negative, it will be placed in the third dial.

Therefore, combining these two coefficients, the more consistent their tonality and their pregnance, the more localized to the centre of representation they are. The computed formula for these coefficients, for each referential criterion, is:

- pregnance index—p*=1/k (a+b);
- tonality index—t*=1/k (a-b);

Table 2-2. Tonality and pregnance coefficients of the identitary social representation

Crt. no.	Referential criteria	a	B	p*	t*
1	S	49	16	.0153	.0303
2	EmV	34	9	.0232	.0400
3	P	53	11	.0156	.0238
4	C	54	56	-.0090	-.5000
5	Ac	27	7	.0294	.0500
6	Cal	18	14	.0312	.2500
7	D	15	17	-.0312	-.0500
8	EvTr	3	68	-.0140	-.0153
9	LR	31	7	.0263	.0416
10	M	33	13	.0217	.0500
11	Fam	67	27	.0106	.0250
12	CatS	11	5	.0625	.1666
13	SfEc	9	2	.0909	.1428
14	Aut	1	16	-.0588	-.0666
15	CatP	8	30	-.0263	-.0370
16	DsP	0	55	-.0181	-.0181
17	Sb	19	0	.0526	.0526
18	Rel	15	9	.0416	.1666
19	Vct	25	3	.0357	.0454
20	Ed	41	9	.0200	.0313

Observation:

- a=frequency of occurrence for the respective referential criteria assessed positively
- b=frequency of occurrence for the respective referential criteria negatively assessed; $k=1 \Leftrightarrow a>=b$ V $k=-1 \Leftrightarrow a<b$.

The results indicate the values of these coefficients, used for the graphical profile of social representation (see Table 2-2 above and Figure 2-5 below).

If we resume the signification of this graphical configuration (see Figure 2-6 below), we can distinguish that the knot of social representation is formed by two poles, constructed around two consistent discursive anchors.

The first pole centres on “family” and what could be integrated in the larger category of “custom” (like “work” and “education”), and confronts “destiny” and “trauma,” generated especially by “political categories” which form the second pole of representation.

The graph suggests the affinity of association between the criteria which are contiguous, generating two distinct classes of similar registers: one full of vitality and engaging, especially informal, and another disengaging, threatening, and preponderantly formal.

If we have to systemize this symbolic confrontation between poles around the including category of “custom” or “trauma,” we should rewrite the symbolic dispute inside the central knot of social representation as shown in the following figures (2-5 and 2-6).

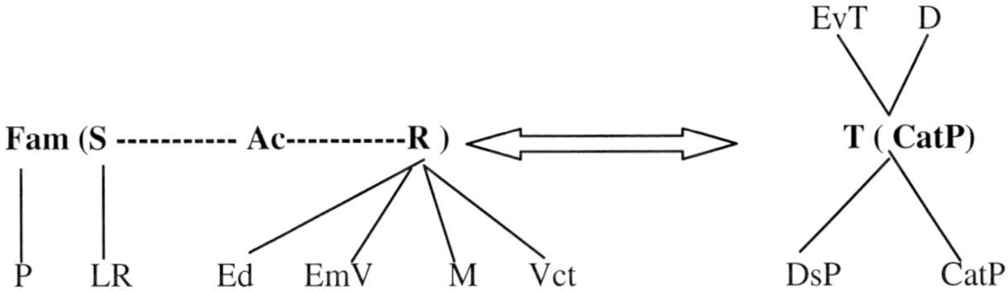

Figure 2-5. Poles of the identitary social representation knot

Other elements that could not be included in the zone circumscribed around these poles have, in general, a conjectural occurrence. For that reason, these categories could be localized inside the peripheral system of representation with the exception of "otherness," which indicates a very low level of tonality but a significant pregnance.

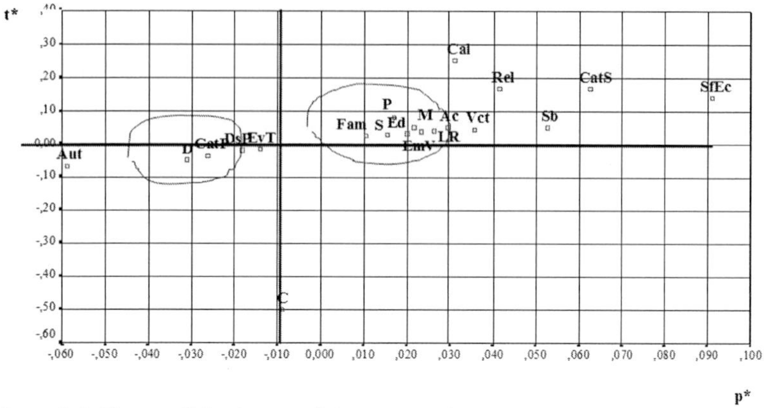

Figure 2-6. Figure of identitary social representation

This also reconfirmed the decisive role assumed by "family," such as the importance of "custom." Thus, the individual and the collective subject could master the discrimination of history and its main protagonists, associated with the political world.

Conclusion

The complexity of such a territory of investigation also imposes an adequate methodology. We have chosen the study, through content analysis, of a sample from the Archive of the Cultural Anthropology and Oral History Group, being aware that we will be able to catch only a tendentious portrait. We have localized three large thematic registers, centred on the individual, community-society and culture, which in turn are grouped around the "self," around the images of "home," the "other," "family," "celebrations," "traumatic events," "political discriminations" and so on. At the same time, we have applied a multilevel value scale to such a discursive thematic destructuring which differentiates between the instrumental and the finality values. If we were to sum up a few of our previous valuations, it would be proper to mention the following:

- From the retrospective discourses, in the thematic area of the "individual," the "self" constructs itself a positive identity, confirming the theories of the social identity, which argue for the decisive role of self-respect in the interpersonal balance and the seeking of a positive social identity within the affiliation group (Tajfel & Turner 1986). Such a strategy is mainly achieved by out-group differentiation, the "other" oscillating between the radical alterity ("it is another world") and total similarity ("they are like us"). It is interesting that in the elaboration of the "other" image, the positive and appreciative features prevail when alterity is described generically, and the critical ones when the "other" becomes an individual presence. Along the discourses, the profile of a traumatic identity is born, which finds its refuge in the nucleus of the family. The "family" is most frequently mentioned in discourses, reuniting, at the same time, most of the positive valuations of all the referential criteria, facing a contorted history, but over which it is capable of projecting a serene light resulting from a superior retrospective understanding which acquires a new meaning. The self-narrative evoked by Gergen (2009) is outlined, conferring coherence to the past and teaching the social actor to look upon the existential drama serenely and to also heal through words.

- At the level of social representation of memorial identity, the "family" references are imposed in a symbolic confrontation with categories associated with "trauma." Thus, the narrative anchors related to "family" become the most influential categories of memorial discourses, representing the core of self-identification in the biographical overview.

References

Abric, J. Cl. (1994). *Représentations sociales et pratiques* [Social and Practical Representations]. Paris: Presses Universitaires de France.

Bertaux, D. (1997). *Le récit de vie* [A Life Story]. Paris: Nathan.

Blumer, H. (1969). *Symbolic interactionism: Perspective and Method*, Englewood: Prentice Hall.

de Rosa, A. S. (2012). Taking stock: a theory with more than half a century of history. In A. S. de Rosa (Ed.), *Social Representations in the "social arena": the theory in contexts faced with "social demand."* New York – London: Routledge.

Elias, N. (1991). *La société des individus* [The Society of Individuals]. Paris: Fayard.

Flament, C. (1995). Structura, dinamica şi transformarea reprezentărilor sociale [Structure, dynamics and transformation of social representations]. In A. Neculau (Ed.), *Psihologia cîmpului social.*

Reprezentările sociale [Psychology of the social field: Social representations] Bucureşti: Ştiinţă şi Tehnică SA. 155-176.

Gavreliuc, A. (2003/2006). *Mentalitate și societate. Cartografii ale imaginarului identitar din Banatul contemporan* [Mentality and society: Mapping the identity imaginary of contemporary Banat]. Timişoara, Romania: West University Press.

Gergen K. & Gergen, M. M. (1988). Narrative and the Self as Relationship. In L. Berkowitz (Ed.), *Advances in Experimental Psychology*. New York, NY: Academic Press.

Gergen, K. (2009). *Relational Being*. New York, NY: Oxford University Press.

Kaufmann, J. Cl. (1998). Interviul comprehensive [Comprehensive Interview]. In Fr. de Singly, Al. Blanchet, A. Gotman, & J. Cl. Kaufmann (Eds.), *Ancheta şi metodele ei: chestionarul, interviul de producere a datelor, interviul comprehensive.* Iaşi: Polirom. 201-310.

Rokeach, M. (1973). *The Nature of Human Values.* New York, NY: Free Press.

Rostaş, Z. (1985). Documentele sociale şi istoria orală [Social Documents and Orl History]. In S. Chelcea (Ed.), *Semnificaţia documentelor sociale*. Bucureşti: Editura Ştiinţifică şi Enciclopedică. 61-77.

Tajfel, H. & Turner, J. C. (1986). The social identity theory of intergroup behaviour. In S. Worchel & W. Austin, (eds.), *Psychology of intergroup relations*, Chicago, MI: Nelson Hall.

Todorov, T. (1998). *Les abus de la mémoire* [Memory Abuse]. Paris: Arléa.

Vultur, S. & Onică, A. (2009). *Memoria salvată (II). Cine salvează o viaţă salvează lumea întreagă* [Saved Memory II : Who Saves a Life Saves the Entire World]. Timişoara: Editura Universității de Vest.

STYLING THE VIRTUAL SELF: CASTELLS AND BAUDRILLARD ON IDENTITIES IN THE NETWORK SOCIETY

ŞTEFAN-SEBASTIAN MAFTEI

Introduction

As the 1990s came to an end the issue of "virtual reality," linked to the rise of the new "information technologies" (Castells 2004) (viz. ARPANET, the internet, etc.), was intensely scrutinised by contemporary sociologists and philosophers alike (Webster 1995; Baudrillard 2003; Castells 1996; 1997; 1998; Turkle 1995; Cerulo 1997; Jones 1997). In the context of the intense globalization of cultures and societies at the end of the twentieth century, and the concomitant development of the global information technologies, the search of the individual for "identity" in the new "network society" (Castells 2004) also came under the spotlight of sociologists.

Castells—When the "Self" Goes Against the "Network"

Castells will define the "network society" (Castells 2004), or the "informational society" (Castells 1994), as a peculiar arrangement of societal relations and social institutions that resulted from the impact of a new form of social communication and organization generated in conjunction with the emergence of the new information technologies. In his 1996 book *Rise of the Network Society*, he does not perceive a deterministic relation with respect to the impact of information technologies upon social movements; he simply describes the advent of a new era from 1969 onwards, marked by a "historical coincidence" by several factors: the informational revolution of the 1960s, the economic crisis of the early 1970s, and the social movements of the 1960s and 70s (1998, 336). He observes the emergence of a new "dominant social structure," the "network society," out of the "interaction" of the processes discussed above, and not out of a deterministic effect of the technology upon society. However, his thesis has been criticized by authors such as Webster (1995, 194 ff.), who concludes that Castells' theory cannot escape the spectre of technological determinism, even if Castells separates capitalist development from the "informational mode" of development. Several times, even Castells himself refers to an "informational technological revolution" preceding, although not determining, all other major structural transformations. In the end, Castells agrees that technology is a key factor in contemporary social change (2004, 8). The informationalist change in the spreading of information and communication, which is a material change in the conditions of their performance, will definitely affect the whole sphere of human society. As such, the "network society" will be defined as "a society whose social structure is made of networks powered by microelectronics-based information and communication technologies" (Ibid., 3).

To Castells, "identity" represents the expression of the "self," either in society or individually. However, the "self" opposes the "network," and this is the main core of his theory about identity in the network society. The reason for this mutual exclusion between the network and the self lies in the nature of the network itself. On one hand, Castells defines the network as a flexible and self-regulating unit, "a set of interconnected nodes … Nodes only exist and function as components of networks. The network is the unit, not the node" (Ibid.). On the other hand, the network works either by exclusion or by inclusion: "Networks work on a binary logic: inclusion/exclusion. Within the network, distance between nodes tends to zero, as networks follow the logic of small worlds' properties … Between nodes in the network and those outside the network distance is infinite, since there is no access unless the program of the network is changed" (Ibid., 4).

This binary feature of the network necessarily produces not just inclusion, but also exclusion. Exclusion is thus a feature built into the network itself. At the social level, the "network society" necessarily fosters exclusion. It creates, as Castells contends, an "informational class" of citizen-employees, and an "underclass" of citizen-employees that are not connected to the nodal points of informationalisation, which are nowadays highly representative for the "commanding heights" of the global economy (Webster 1995, 200). The network itself draws a very definite line between the informationalised and the non-informationalised classes.

Consequently, the network divide produces, at a general level, social fragmentation. At the individual level, this network divide alienates the individual from their own personal identity, deeply embedded in their local culture, since it forces them to take part to the new, global, networked, *laissez-faire* culture. According to Castells, these global networks create a global culture where the network itself structures "production, consumption, communication and power" (Castells 2004, 23). In the new dominant logic of the network society, globalization is for the most part "exclusive." Despite its ideological claims, the "global" may and will exclude that which is not considered "global," that which does not fit, according to Castells, the impetus of self-expansion in the development of the informational global networks. "Fragmentation," as a multi-faceted phenomenon of the global world, is built into the system. This is happening precisely because, according to its own dominant logic of self-expansion, the reconfiguring capacity inscribed in the process of networking allows the programs governing every network to search for valuable additions everywhere and to incorporate them, while bypassing and excluding those territories, activities, and people that have little or no value for the performance of the tasks assigned to the network.

The global will, in effect, "overwhelm the local, unless the local becomes a node in alternative global networks" (Ibid.). Following Castells, the self is thus fragmented by the globalizing tendencies of the new, global, informationalised culture.

Identity, mainly informed by local culture, language, religion and customs, when forced to live in a globalized world, reacts in its own peculiar way to social and cultural fragmentation. Facing intense pressure from the globalized world of "wealth, power and images," the self reacts by "regrouping around primary identities: religious, ethnic, territorial, national" (Castells 1996, 3). Sensing the destructuring trends in administration, the "delegitimation of institutions," the political crisis of legitimation, the ephemerity of culture and values, identity, deeply rooted in its local culture, becomes, as Castells admits, the "only source of meaning." In the network society, the self-asserting, dominating logic of the network, fostering a new universalism, is counterbalanced by the resistance of the self: "When the Net switches off the self, the self, individual or collective, constructs its meaning without global, instrumental reference: the process of disconnection becomes reciprocal, following the refusal by the excluded of the one-sided logic of structural domination and social exclusion" (Ibid., 24).

Moreover, if identity is defined, according to Castells, by mutual exclusion between the internet and the self, this exclusion does not generate a passive resistance from the self only. The aggressive, dominating force of globalization is countered, in Castells' view, by a no less aggressive counteraction of the self (either individual or social). In fact, this polarization only deepens the differences and heightens the tensions between the globalized culture and localized, particularized selves. What we have today in the world, Castells contends, is not a global culture, but a struggle between a networked culture advancing its own ideology and a "multiplicity of local selves" (Castells 2004, 39). With the advancement of globalization in the world, this struggle is becoming acutely violent:

> Our societies are increasingly structured around a bipolar opposition between the Net and the self … And when communication breaks down … social groups and individuals become alienated from each other, and see the other as a stranger, eventually as a threat. In this process, social fragmentation spreads, as identities become more specific and increasingly difficult to share. (Castells 1996, 3–4)

Why does Castells associate the self's search for identity in a network society with a grim vision of radical self-assertion, violence and sectarianism? After all, the "self exists in social life." Therefore, "the social sources of self make subjectivity possible because the person's experience of feelings, images, and interpretations emerges and takes on meaning through social interaction" (Charmaz 2007, 4165). According to Mead (Ibid.), the self is "reflexive" and "socially structured," and is both a social process and a social object. In addition, it is "simultaneously social and subjective." It reacts as a "social structure," and it "differs according to the social situation." Particularly, a certain situation "calls forth *a* self because people's varied situations lead to possessing different selves." According to Mead, the self develops "in active response to what occurs around it. This response may consist of internalization, adaptation, innovation, or resistance" (Ibid., 4166). Mead's vision is that of a quasi-organic self, reacting not only to stimuli, but also to social, cultural or economic inputs. The self is thus not only social, but also proteic, creative, and, moreover, multi-faceted. It is both a process and an object, a self-made but not self-sufficient entity. It is, in a way, a "stylized" self, if we may borrow a term from aesthetics, or, better yet, an "aesthetic" self, if aesthetics is willing to widen its boundaries (Seppä 2004). We will return to this topic later.

To answer the question about Castells' identity, we should bring forth two issues. First is the fact that the network is, in itself, exclusionary, as Castells argues. This thesis seems like an offshoot of the Marxist view about technology or the machine as an instrument for the alienation of the human from itself and the selves of others. As far as other, more recent studies have shown, the globalized network of communication technologies, mostly the internet with its integrated capabilities of communication, is doing exactly the opposite. It is not alienating one person's sense of the self from another's sense of the self, but fostering communication between the individual selves, and probably reframing our sense of identity. According to some authors (Bakardjieva 2005; Cerulo 1997), "new communication technologies" (NCT) not only enable "new communication formats … creating new environments for self-development and communication … presenting new opportunities for collective affiliation and mobilization," but really "change the backdrop against which identity is constructed," thus reshaping our whole sense of identity (Cerulo 1997, 397). NCTs can even foster a "self-conscious collective agency" (Ibid., 396).

Second, there is the manner in which Castells sees the concept of identity. According to him, identity is always exclusionary, as "the process by which a social actor recognizes itself and constructs meaning primarily on the basis of a given cultural attribute or set of attributes, to the exclusion of a broader reference to other social structures" (Castells 1996, 22). In other words, the self always defines itself as representing a set of values which is in opposition to another set of values. Throughout the world, Castells observes "the increasing distance between globalization and identity, between the Net and the self" (Ibid.). On the other hand, he admits that "while information systems and networking augment human powers of organization and integration, they simultaneously subvert the traditional Western concept of a separate, independent subject" (Ibid., 23). This explains his view of a self which is much related to the traditional view of the "independent subject." He thus admits the view of an independent identity, permeated by a set of values that excludes others.

Nevertheless, provided that the self, with its sense of identity, is not an essentialistic construct, explainable only as an independent subjective entity, but, in line with contemporary sociology, a more fluctuating, more social, and more inter-dependent reality, studies have shown that NCT, particularly the internet, are not only elements which contribute to identity-building, shaping new "virtual selves" with "virtual identities" (DiMicco & Millen 2007; Behm-Morawitz 2013), but are, as objects, relevant to "identity-building interactions" when "media objects become a viable 'other' in the building of the self, and they outline the ways in which human-to-machine relationships mirror purely human relationships" (Cerulo 1997, 399). Hence, we cannot "reify a single, static notion of the self" instead of "theorizing the multiplicity of selves and their processual nature" (Charmaz 2007, 4167).

This is not to say that there is no continuity of one's self throughout life. According to Charmaz (2007), new theories assert that there is a difference between a process of the self and a stable structure, which is "the self concept." The fact is that while the processes of the self goes on and off, "meanings about the self last." People always seek to define themselves, and this act of defining the self includes "definitions of self, sentiments, values, judgments, through which a person describes himself or herself." This is the stable part of the "enduring self." However, this endurance depends on the self's own response to the reactions of others (Ibid., 4167). The self is thus not above the social. At best, it creates the social by affirming itself, creatively, inside the "net" of the social relationships of power and, thus, in a certain way, by resisting the networks of social power while at the same time transforming them. The self is thus not only about "resistance," but also about processes of "reconstruction," "development" and "transformation," even in cases of adult selves. There is hence no "asocial, reductionist and static self" in the majority of today's theories about the self (Ibid., 4168).

Virtual Aesthetics of the Self

The self and its identity are not above the social, and are more or less in a state of continuous transformation. In the above, we have raised the issue of the aesthetic self, posing serious challenges to the modern notion of the aesthetic (Seppä 2004). Although it seems like an offshoot of the Enlightenment's idea of the human, which envisions the enlightened human being as the result of civilization, culture and beauty, far from its natural, brutish state, the idea of the "aesthetics of the self" is not easily discernible in the atmosphere of early and late modernity. However, aestheticism has for a long time been a part of modern literary aesthetics, in the works of Baudelaire and Wilde. Directed against modern materialism and modern capitalist relations, by emphasizing the cult of artistic disinterestedness and the authentic life-style of the artist, the aestheticist *culte du moi*, incarnated in the modern dandy, is a modern attitude characterised by the "willingness to make one's body, behaviour, passions and existence a work of art" (Seppä 2004). However, it does not fit the "high modernity" pattern established by the authors, such as Kant, who shared a rationalistic, universalizable view of the human of the Enlightenment. In the aestheticist culture of the nineteenth century, however, beauty was not an abstraction, but involved the very life of the contingent individual. Beauty lies in the individual's psyche, in their gestures, manners, life-style, body, clothing, etc. In Baudelaire's sense, to be modern is an act of personal, individual choice, not an acceptance of a universal norm. To quote Oscar Wilde, our duty as aestheticists is to "be as artificial as possible," that is, one should "either be a work of art, or wear a work of art" (in Seppä 2004). Moreover, morality itself should be grounded "on the order of the beautiful," as Baudelaire dictated (Seppä 2004). In a way, this is a work of "*inventing* yourself," by creating a "personal aesthetics of the self," and not of "*discovering*" yourself. Truth, which lies only in beauty, viz. in the contingent act of making yourself beautiful, is not a predetermined notion. Truth is a question of performance, and it is a contingent truth dependent on an elusive, fluctuant, transitory beauty (Seppä 2004). Following Scott Lash and Jonathan Friedman's distinction between "high modernity" and "low modernity," Seppä considers that the aestheticists embraced an aesthetics of the "low," being particularly interested in melting the aesthetics of the "body," "affectiveness" and the "everyday life" into an aesthetic doctrine that emphasized those aspects of subjectivity that were lacking in Kant's aesthetics. In her account of the relationship between the early aestheticists and their influence on late authors, such as Foucault, Seppä establishes three major differences between modern Kantian subject of aesthetics and the Baudelairean "aesthetics of the self." The first is that aestheticism sees the modern individual as determined not by the "universally valid structures of reason," but by their own self-creation or self-emancipation. The second is that aestheticism emphasizes the aesthetic education of the body and the discovery of its sexuality. The aestheticist identity, as we find out in Baudelaire, Wilde and Foucault, is closely related to the body as the seat of identity. The third difference involves the idea of historical progress, which the aestheticists denied, insisting that "modern aesthetics is not rooted in the individual's public usage of reason" (Seppä 2004).

It is obvious that there are considerable differences between an aestheticized image of the self and the perception of subjectivity in modern aesthetics. Firstly, as Seppä contends, the so-called "aesthetic practices" of the self are not limited to aesthetics, but are also a part of a person's ethical and political conduct. The aesthetic self-empowerment is thus not limited to the realm of modern aesthetic experience. Secondly, the way in which the aesthetics of the self envisions the "aesthetic" subject is different: the aesthetic subject is not the universalizable subject of Kant's philosophy, but a concrete subject which manifests themselves through gestures, passions, bodily image and individual appearance, shaping for themselves their own "individual style." This is the concrete, individualized subject of aesthetics, deliberately cultivating its own, self-styled image. Thirdly, this subject's identity is not fixed, it is performative and transitory. There is no fixed, abstractly or naturally grounded notion of the self and its identity (Ibid.).

The modern dream of individuality, viz. of the subject's authenticity and disinterestedness, thus survives even in the most concrete aestheticized descriptions of the self. However, Foucault's writings on this subject address some theoretical concerns regarding this new notion of the self in late modernity. First, Foucault challenges the view that this aestheticized self cannot be, in turn, subjected to criticism and transgressions, and thus altered. The second challenge is more serious, referring to the alleged independence of the aestheticized subject in late modernity, because some would agree that even if the self does not establish a fixed identity, it can still act as an independent self. Although Foucault addresses the issues of self-control many times, regarding the self-empowerment of the concrete subject, he remains altogether skeptical about the subject's power of emancipating itself from the "normalizing" practices of post-industrial societies. Thus, even if the self-emancipated subject can sometimes be aestheticized as a subject of political struggle, there is still the risk that the emancipation might be a false one, and that the individual self will crack under the pressure of the normalization powers of societies. One could take, for example, the subject of the "docile bodies" that are aestheticized, i.e. embellished, normalized, under the current "aesthetic practices of appearance," shaping one's body into stereotypical beauty patterns and fashion ideals in aesthetic surgery clinics (Seppä 2004). In this context, "aestheticism" can convey a shallow meaning to the processes of self-aestheticizing. How are we to differentiate between cultural docility and authentic aesthetic self-emancipation? (Groys 2009)

The same reading may be applied to virtual identity in our networked world. As already shown, there is an aesthetics of the virtual self going on in the virtual environments (Bakardjieva 2005; DiMicco & Miller 2007; Behm-Morawitz 2013; Gottschalk 2010; Bloustien & Wood 2013). I will define "virtual self" as the self representing itself through and being represented through computer/internet technology in the social world. I therefore consider that the virtual self is an application of the aestheticization of the self as a self-image in the virtual environments. It is an application mainly because it is a self that is not a product, but a creative process. The virtual self refers not to an abstract self, but to a contingent self that is reflecting itself, as an image, in the virtual world in roughly the same way a person would see themselves, or would be seen in a mirror. The virtual self is thus the internet (computer), a mediated self (Bakardjieva 2005, 65 ff.). As well as in the case of aestheticization's described above, the virtual self can bring forth either an empowered image or a weaker, disempowered image of the self. I would also refer here, as Bakardjieva does, to the notion of "self-production," which destroys alienation related to technology and restores the identity to the individual. Bakardjieva also contends that the virtual self may be included in an everyday life critique of human existence: "even if an individual's involvement in the process of social production taken in its economic sense is marked by alienation, a whole range of diverse productive activities still remain open at the level of everyday life for her free and creative engagement" (Ibid., 53). Here, "everyday life" is defined as "the terrain in which the individual is an actor physically and mentally involved in producing, in its widest sense, the social world and her own self" (Ibid., 57). Nevertheless, different from the self-aestheticized concrete individual, the networked self is more prone to being integrated into a "community model" of communication. In other words, it is possible for the self-creation of the virtual self to be more dependent on social communication through the internet than on the personal, individual strategies of self-creation. The sense of the self as a seat of authenticity and aesthetic disinterestedness is starting to vanish in the virtual world.

Baudrillard's "Virtual"

A very concrete virtual aestheticization of the self is taking place on the Internet platform Second Life (Behm-Morawitz 2013; Gottschalk 2010; Bloustien & Wood 2013). Here, the conceptual boundaries between the virtual and the real life of the self, the distinction between the public and the private, seem to fade away. Second Life is based on the "avatar," which is the virtual simulation of the individual's self in real life. Studies (Behm-Morawitz 2013) show that the "avatar" is not only a virtual simulation—it acts precisely as a virtual self, stimulating "one's cognition, behaviour and well being." There is thus a construction of the offline self through the "avatar," which is similar to an aestheticization process. This is created by the phenomenon of "presence," which is explained as a "perceptual illusion of nonmediation," produced by the human "extended consciousness" which "allows one to suspend disbelief and experience the virtual as a possible reality" (Ibid., 120). This instead generates the phenomenon of "self-presence," which allows the subjects to experience "their virtual self as if they were their actual" (Ibid., 121).

This is precisely the point emphasized by Baudrillard in his theory about "virtuality" (Baudrillard 2003; Smith 2010). He names this the "post-human dimension," at the moment when the virtual:

> replaces the actual as the primary mode by which we conceptualize and experience reality. Humans have become virtualized—immersed within digital circuits of instant and excessive information technologies—to the point where we can no longer maintain a critical distance from the cyberspaces that surround us. (Ibid., 16)

However, Baudrillard is a critical author, and is neither a supporter of aestheticism nor a prophet of the post-human. He contends that the internet merely "simulates a free mental space, a space of freedom and discovery" (Ibid.). Baudrillard explains the virtual as a semiologist. The virtual is an "integral reality," a world saturated with signifiers, "codes." In this logic, the post-human internet reality offers no way out of the total domination of the reality by the sign (Ibid., 34). The virtual is "that which takes the place of the real" entirely. It is "the final solution of the real in so far as it both accomplishes the world in its definitive reality and marks its dissolution" (Baudrillard 2003, 39–40). He also talks about the "third-order simulation," which is the moment when simulation appears by itself, without any reference to the simulated thing. The virtual is a copy without an original. It has lost its point of reference outside itself. It is a fully closed world of signs. It is not a copy, it is really a "clone" of the offline world (2010, 237). At this stage, there is no difference between the real and the virtual, if there ever was one. Moreover, if the effect of the virtual is a total effect, then all reference to the sign as sign, to the "symbolic dimension" or to "illusion," dies. There is no longer a representation: "in the sphere of the Virtual … nothing is representable … neither distance nor a critical or aesthetic gaze: there is total immersion … not of the order of representation, but of decoding and visual consumption … it is impossible to work back from them to some tangible reality" (in Smith, 2010, 238). In other works, he sees the virtual's detachment from the real as a possibility for the emancipation of the subject from a thinking which is guided by objectivity and purposiveness. The outcome is not clear—technology may be either liberating or destructive (2010, 239). Nevertheless, Baudrillard poses serious challenges to theorists of the cybersociety.

Conclusion

The fate of "identity" in Baudrillard's theory however remains uncertain. Identity can be either an effect of a total domination of the virtual or it can alter the effects of alienation and reification through an emancipatory strategy which regards the discovery of an emancipatory power of the "objective irony" concerning the total domination of the virtual. In other words, the total disappearance of the "real" into the "virtual" may have the opposite, emancipatory effect of creating disbelief in the passive audience. However, according to Groys (2009), aestheticization in the virtual world, not only in the arts, is a puzzling issue. In the end, aestheticization is corrosive, since it carries with its justifications the same theoretical puzzles that have baffled aestheticians for almost three centuries, and extends these puzzles to the political and ethical values of a person's action. If aestheticization is authentic, how can we establish its "authenticity?" Also, if the ethical or political emancipation of the individual is also a matter of aestheticization, then what constitutes a correct ethical or political choice in terms of aestheticization? Through his criticism, Groys stresses the need for establishing new aesthetic, ethical and political boundaries for the new "aestheticized" strategies of the self.

Acknowledgement

This work was supported by a grant of the Romanian National Authority for Scientific Research, CNCS—UEFISCDI, project number PN-II-ID-PCE-2011-3-1010.

References

Bakardjieva, M. (2005). *Internet Society. The Internet in Everyday Life*. London: Sage.

Baudrillard, J. (2003). *Passwords*. London: Verso.

Behm-Morawitz, E. (2013). Mirrored selves: The influence of self-presence in a virtual world on health, appearance, and wellbeing. *Computers in Human Behavior 29*: 119-128.

Bloustien, G. F. & Wood, D. (2013). Face, Authenticity, Transformations and Aesthetics. *Second Life, Body & Society 19 (1)*: 52-81.

Castells, M. (1994). European Cities, the Informational Society, and the Global Economy. *New Left Review 204*: 18-32.

—. (1996). *The Information Age: Economy, Society and Culture.Volume 1: The Rise of the Network Society*. Oxford: Blackwell.

—. (1997). *The Information Age: Economy, Society and Culture. Volume 2: The Power of Identity*. Oxford: Blackwell.

—. (1998). *The Information Age: Economy, Society and Culture 3: End of Millennium.* Oxford: Blackwell.

Castells, M. (Ed.). (2004). *The Network Society. A Cross-Cultural Perspective*. Cheltenham: Edward Elgar.

Cerulo, K. (1997). Identity Construction. New Issues, New Directions. *Annual Review of Sociology 23*: 385-409.

Charmaz, K. (2007). Self. In G. Ritzer (Ed.), *The Blackwell Encyclopedia of Sociology*. Oxford: Blackwell: 4165-4169.

DiMicco, J. M. & Millen, D. R. (2007). Identity management: multiple presentations of self in Facebook. *GROUP '07: Proceedings of the 2007 international ACM conference on Supporting group work*: 383-386.

Gottschalk, S. (2010). The Presentation of Avatars in Second Life: Self and Interaction in Social Virtual Spaces. *Symbolic Interaction 33 (4)*: 501-525.

Groys, B. (2009). Self-design and Aesthetics Responsibility. *E-Flux. Journal 7 (06)*. Online at: http://www.e-flux.com/journal/self-design-and-aesthetic-responsibility.

Jones, S. G. (Ed.). (1997). *Virtual Culture: Identity and Communication in Cybersociety*. Beverly Hills, CA: Sage.

Seppä, A. (2004). Foucault, Enlightenment and the Aesthetics of the Self, *Contemporary Aesthetics 2*. Online: http://www.contempaesthetics.org/newvolume/pages/article.php?articleID=244&searchstr=Foucault%2C+Enlightenment+and+the+Aesthetics+of+the+Self.

Smith, R. G. (Ed.). (2010). *The Baudrillard Dictionary*. Edinburgh: Edinburgh University Press.

Turkle, S. (1995). *Life on the Screen: Identity in the Age of the Internet*. London: Secker & Warburg.

Webster, F. (1995). *Theories of the Information Society*. London: Routledge.

IDENTITARY COMPLICITIES IN THE VISUAL ERA

ȘTEFANIA BEJAN

Introduction

The positive connotation of the challenge motivates thinkers to look at post-modernity from a daring perspective in the "narrow circle" of the field of mass communication. Being "acclimatized" to the debates about what it looks like, "what it does" and "towards who it's heading," the era following the modern period cannot sustain, in the full serenity of conscience, that the subject of discussion is clear, that the dating is clear, and that the prospects are easy to indicate, eventually, pressing the (unspoken) question—what comes after post-modernity? (Logic "knows" that two negations generate an affirmation, therefore, in the absence of an established expression regarding post-post-modernity, naturally it would follow—in fact, there would be a return towards—modernity). Bizarre, unbelievable, necessary?! Let us not lose sight, though, that the "unifying portrait" of "pre-post-modernity" has been anachronistic for decades, which changes everything. In other words, it leaves room for some "sidelong glances," and is suspicious in the profitable sense of the term; how can one "dissect" post-modernity (in this case, the communicational one), if not enough time has elapsed to "weigh" the mark (the stakes, "the tasks") of modernity within this professional field? In Brunner's opinion, the contemporary society is marked by hedonism, consisting of winners, due to the desire of the ego/subject to succeed in life. Subsumed by the ideology of management, of efficiency, this strategy implies the possibility of the subject to project themselves in the future, to "plan" their life. While the ego calculates, the self opposes, wanting to take advantage of the offer of life here and now (Brunner 2000, 41–43). The idolatry of the present means, according to Brunner, a terrible hatred towards time; to feel victorious because the temporal distance between the time you aim for something and when you succeeded has comprised the immediate instant. Living in a society that isn't characterized by patience, which doesn't respect the pleasure of waiting, the ego/contemporary subject "gives up declining the past and imagining the future. This subject too rushed doesn't know that he is losing his time hurrying" (Brunner 2000, 49). In the order of gains there is, alongside career, money and material goods, more and more free time, which in recent years the person has "spent" having fun (treating everything in a relaxed manner, investing in an industry of entertainment, seeking social recognition or identity building on the pattern of entertainment), because "the hatred towards time means fear of empty time." The emergence of "sports-entertainment" and "chewing gum" television announces the fear of boredom, of too many unoccupied hours, which you don't know how to "kill." Brunner speaks of "the resistance to the amplification of an available, yet meaningless time," and the interest/toil in finding a convenient manner to choose/establish one's identity. Until recently, the identitary markers were called (excepting origin, race, ethnicity, religion and so on) work, profession and enterprise (it is not to be understood that the author lays any blame on work and an increased quantity of leisure. However, he does not hesitate to declare the existence of a "social chaos" arising from the inability of beneficially occupying free time). Brunner's apocalyptic vision contains references to a teleocratic strategy in which the obscenity of the ego has no limits, given the availability of stars and regular people to "strip" in front of the viewer, and which can be seen everywhere. Nothing is kept intimate (private) any longer; everything must be told, shown, and revealed in and by the mass media. Those who do not "process" their image are destined to fail as an individual or part of an organisation. The perfecting of this communicational logic is attributed to the political area where "Tartuffe and the sophists dominate." Brunner loudly declares that we are dealing with a communication "front of the persuasion of the masses, of the manipulation through political propaganda, of the wooden language … of the seduction specific to advertising, of the panoptic conception of social control" (Brunner 2000, 54).

Methods

The documentary analysis and interviews with renowned or academic intellectuals easily reveal, in a controversial manner, the temptation of the urgent (sometimes definitive) placement in the online environment. Connecting to social networks, achieving the postmodern communicational status, and the increasing influence of self-promotion, at the risk of challenging the multiple avatar-masks, gains more and more popularity, even if they seem like part of a new conformism. The conditions, exigencies and dangers of positioning in the virtual environment are known and, as long as they don't depart fundamentally from those of the classicized-obsolete communication, at least partially, they can be assumed. To communicate constantly, to behave yourself, to search for many friends, to not post untruths, to enjoy power and "likes," to demand communication that is "direct, short, to the point" (Bădău 2011, 159), is to notice honestly that not all interlocutors (including virtual friends) who respect the rules of genuine dialogue represent the height of innovation.

Discussions and Results

Displaying, with premeditation, the mask of innocence, we can advance a tripartition of the challenges "brought" to the arena of the academic community:

- Positive
- At the boundary between beneficial and damaging
- Negative.

The first would cover: de-massification, the blurring of the boundaries between the different media, the interactivity as a consequence of the "administration" by the media of social relations, the individuality specific to the contemporary era, a novel form of the reality (and the practice it circumscribes); the rule of either-or (maybe, neither-nor), in the median area would find its place; the democratization of knowledge, a new type of socializing, the resistance of the traditional media, the evolution of mass communication according to the rules practiced over centuries, the domination of a harmony occurring, paradoxically, from a-synchrony; and subject to harsh criticism for alleged unwanted effects, in the long term, are the entertainment which becomes a strategy governing the editorial policies in mass media and the imperialism of the internet, which are difficult to impede in a mimetic society.

Bringing to attention the socio-cultural "place" of the means of communication intended for a "public" that is anonymous, heterogeneous, spatially dispersed (yet "driven" by desires, interests that are imaginary, as in the comfortable majority), the phrases that express the identity and mission of the press mentally persist (actors of the public space, technological devices, power factors, cultural industries, instances producing discourses, relays of information, vectors of information) (Drăgan 2007, 330).

Depicting the model of spatio-temporal extension of John B. Thompson, from *The Media and Modernity: A Social Theory of the Media*, by the sociological treatment (transmitting messages-evaluating effects), and by virtue of the language sciences ("process of production and interpretation of the symbolic forms revealed through their discursive manifestation"), the hermeneutics "targeting" mass media give a clear verdict of symbolic power (as found in the British Cultural Studies School, by Pierre Bourdieu). The hypostases of the press in its evolution of more than four centuries at present has echoes of the European Middle Ages. It is a *pillar* of the building of modernity, a *miracle* of the twentieth century (when the world doesn't remain exclusively re-presented by the media, but it becomes "saturated" and "transfigured"), and finally the *curse* of the twenty-fist century (given the impact on the clear direction of the future of humanity) (Drăgan 2007, 330).

"The creation of new forms of action and interaction in the social world," as well as "new ways of exercising power, which are no longer related to living together in a common space" prevent, through Thompson's "voice," the radical change of the nature of power in general and "practicing" power from other social fields (political, economic and so on), since communication can only be the "victim" of contextualisation. This can explain typologies such as Balle's (independent, broadcasting, intercommunication media) or Fiske's (presentation, re-presentation, mechanical media), but also the well-known circular pattern (Katz, Gurevitch, Haas), having at the "start" the needs and motivations of the consumers' inclination towards certain channels of communication, along with the preferences of the public and the satisfactions offered by the press. The similarities of any medium with two others in proximity make it easy to fill the absence, no matter what is represented of the media, by taking over the functions (for instance, cinematography "resembles" the books and the television; the newspapers—the books and the radio; television—radio and cinematography, etc.). In other words, after the needs "solved" preponderantly by a certain channel of mass communication, we can "count" the vicinities that are subject to the invoked circular pattern of the media.

The historic "path" of the professional field in discussion has been marked by four "milestones": the increase in the population's educational level, the massification of information, the diversification of channels and the perfecting of techniques. As a result, at the end of the second millennium we find, in fact, the same job only operating with more and more sophisticated tools. Besides, an "invasion" of non-professionals ready to compete with the specialists in the construction and dissemination of the public message sparked, at one point, the fear that we assist a true "death of journalism" (Agnès 2011, 32). (An atypical "exit," certainly, since cameras and mobile phones with applications create "journalists," and users of numerous websites represent clear sources of information). We will have, Agnès opinates, following the model of "participatory democracy" from the political world, "participatory information" ("civic journalism"). It is appropriate to point out that in the online environment rules of deontology aren't "played"; in other words, credibility no longer has the importance of the surplus value from the traditional media! The natural interrogation regards the capacity of interactivity (Baudrillard 2002, 176–180): "Video, interactive screens, multimedia, Internet, virtual reality—we are threatened from all sides by interactivity" (Lovink 2004, 16) to supply the exigency of credibility that we were used to (at least, at the theoretical level). To rephrase—if the internet represents a postmodern form of imperialism, then whose kingdom, which imperator, who conquers whom and, especially, how: "by intercepting messages, through the suspicious use of databases, by the cunningness of attracting children in dangerous informational-entertaining areas?" (Manovich 2001, 27–48) does it invoke traits such as automaticity, modularity, numeric representation, and genuine character.

Re-analyzing the "look" on NTIC, we will doubt, perhaps, the optimism of technophiles (the technological progress brings about a better world), we will criticize the pessimism of technophobes (for which the domination of technologies determines the addiction of the consumer and the shaping of society in patterns that are strictly technical), or—why not?—we will stand in doubt, asking ourselves whether the humanistic values are in crisis, and, still, who would now represent "the centre of the world," the human or technology.

Following Soriano (*Zero-One and the Infinite: A Humanism Without the Human?*), Ghiu resorts to the anatomy of the "Manifest for the Arrival of the New Man," which calms the exaggerated enthusiasm of the technophiles through some arguments with ironic shading: (a) science and technology promote peace and well-being; (b) the network cancels space, time, limits, opening the cultures "captive" in their own anachronistic forms; (c) the same network protects the memory, favouring the unlimited access to infinite databases; (d) the cultural-intellectual inequalities disappear; (e) the synthetic identities, freely consented and whenever revisable appear; (f) "perfectly porous virtual communities" are created; (g) the new human refuses their individualism, becoming "virtually together-with-all-the-others" and releases themselves from the durable belonging to stable and closed communities that constrained them; (h) the personal memory narrows, favouring the disappearance of the annoying intrapersonal communication; (i) the network sends into history the institutional hierarchies which maintained inequalities of all sorts; (j) the combination of genetic engineering with computer science finally gives the postmodern human the opportunity to dominate their genetic heritage (towards immortality?!); (k) the mobile-immobile branching of any human being in an incommensurable availability is facilitated; and (l) the anti-social attitude of self-isolation through reading, praying or meditation is discouraged (Ghiu 2002, 77). Those traditionally attached to the values of modernity (including what regards mass communication) hardly resist the prevention of a new media critic, for whom "the virtual doesn't only affect and attack 'the actuality,' but the virtual itself," since the character of the media as a "second ideology" supports metaphors from the family of words of the virtual, but "the so-called contemporary virtual stimulates and mocks the virtual truth, paralyzes and corrupts the "spectral" structure, ruining it and pushing it to become something else. This way, "the spectre is haunting itself against itself, and comes to be haunted by its metaphysical 'avatar,' so by its own 'being,' with which he had been mistaken for" (Ghiu 2002, 19–20).

According to Lovink, the danger of the disappearance of the "guinea pig" before the crystallization of some value judgements lies ahead in the area of techno-cultural studies. Taking Silver (2000, 19) seriously with the staging of popular cyberculture, cybercultural studies and cybercultural critical studies, the author focuses on the notion of "virtual communities as social networks" and "suggests" the reflection of the contemporary society in the said networks (including anticipations-incarnations of some novel forms of social interaction) (Lovink 2004, 15).

Seeking a sense of the profoundly motivating statement: "The online environment generates another manner of socialization," we bring to attention the point of view expressed by Rasa:

> There are few people who see in the Internet a space of self expression. Most of them aren't aware of the potential of this "new realm." If the dominating attitude is consumption, and not contributing or building, sooner or later, after the 'gold rush' ends, people will find that these "new realms" are empty. (Lovink 2004, 198)

Putting the issue of the independent media "under the microscope" democratically brings it together with the online communication environment. Arthur Kroker criticizes "the new electronic, invisible belligerence" of Europe, intrinsically dependent on "the bitter division of the world in virtual meat and supplementary meat," suggesting the birth of an absolute distrust, formulated this way: "Don't trust the Internet and especially our *site*" (Lovink 2004, 38).

Does the internet serve democracy (cultivating its participatory hypostasis)? Fidler states that, in the opinion of many *users*, the network of the networks represents a "vehicle" that is more profitable to free speech and public debate than the previous media. The example of the voters from the USA at the presidential elections from 2006 via the internet supports the idea of the power (even only hypothetically) of the internet over the opinion leaders, the leaders from the political environment, etc., albeit only by virtue of the age of the electoral "wave" freshly appearing in the "ring" of decision-making (Fidler 2004, 98). The author considers the impossibility of applying the features and rules of traditional media at the level of the "virtual universes" to be wrong. The principles of "survival" and "delayed adoption" justify the functioning of new media in the logic of the "expansion" of the already "outdated" sisters (although some of them have not yet had a decade of functioning). The rhythm becomes alert (but not surprising) in the progress of communicational technologies, but the "lessons" of the past don't disappear by themselves, and therefore we relive the control crisis from the beginning of the nineteenth century, the rapid industrialization generating the need for an accordingly social feedback, and the informatization with its exigencies of storage, processing and dissemination of information. The third mediamorphosis invoked by Fidler involves the radical transformation of the "human notions of distance, time and even reality," thanks to the new media arisen and instituted to meet the opportunity and the need of some users circumscribed to the "mediamorphic process" (Fidler 2004, 99-100).

Let us not ignore the advantages of a new type of social-communicational harmony, regarding the a-synchronicity of the possession of the new media message, giving at least the illusion of the independence and freedom of the user in "contacting" and managing the contents at its will. Simultaneously transmitted to the "de-massificated," but received according to temporal preferences by the individual-consumer, the media discourses recall the binomial order-disorder (succession-simultaneity) into question. On the other hand, the hyper-reality leading to techniques and powers of simulating reality can be decrypted in the key of a surprisingly pleasant manner of building realities as fragments, in the purest Baudrillardian logic of post-modernity (the game with the fragments, the author of *The Consumer Society: Myths and Strucures* said, is all we have left).

Finally, the concern that entertainment—becoming a strategy of the last decades' media—would be diffused-consumed in enormous quantities, at the request of the postmodern consumer, seems justified insofar as the "lack of measure" would animate the majority, diverting (from the perspective of conscience and daily social obligations) the human of the era, perfectly adapted, from a costly agenda.

With roots in the Latin *idem* (similarity, continuity), identity (according to the Explanatory Dictionary of the Romanian Language—perfect similarity; dataset through which a person identifies themselves; alike; exactly; the same as) is regarded by psycho-sociologists by its built, invented character. Goffman & Berger claim that identity is clearly "conferred, sustained and transformed socially." According to James & Mead, the self "unfolds" on two levels: "I"—connoisseur, interior, subjective—and "Me," known, exterior, socially determined (the determination is defined as a process of appointing, placing the man in socially constructed categories). Foucault finds the discourse to be the true nest of the sense of identity, since "the raw material of identity is formed within the discourses, is assumed by an individual who is situated inside of them." The French author believes the human being is responsible for wearing more identities, provided that the various discourses give rise to the specific/divergent positions of identity (male, engineer, generous) and, at the same time, the multiple identities held, which depend on always different social practices, are linked to wider identitary structures (class, gender, race, sexual preferences). In different circumstances, the identities of the same person interact, which explains a certain behaviour, a certain social position, arising from the combination of race, ethnicity, gender, etc.

On this trajectory, the hybridization of cultural identities, the movement and mixture of different cultures resulting in a mosaic identity, is reached. Psychoanalysts explain the identity socially retrieved through the reflection of the individual, even since birth, in someone's eyes. From the self-identification of the infant in the mother's eyes, the narcissistic strategy bases all subsequent identifications of the being for socialization. According to Jacques Lacan, the prolonged report with the visual field can appear as an alienated (off-centre) experience, but also as a rupture between an "ideal ego" (exterior) and the already interiorized "ideal of the ego."

The identitary picture exposed by sociologists has two faces: an optimistic one and a pessimistic one. The first is circumscribed to the modern world and has the advantage of the rise of individuality, along with the possibility to choose from different identities (which leads to the idea of self-realization independent from tradition, religion and culture in general), hence the taste for flexibility, difference and understanding of oneself. The pessimistic version depicts a mass society characterized by estrangement, lack of meaning, lack of delimitation between self and culture, selfishness and self-integration. (It is stated that in modern sociology there isn't a clear concept of identity, but the vague meaning of the term refers to four figures: [1] someone's self-awareness; [2] ideas and feelings regarding oneself; [3] identity through socialization, when we interiorize the social roles that we hold and the expectations regarding them; [4] identity as the sum of the elements presented to us during socialization or in the practice of different social roles). We shall ask ourselves, along with the famous author of stigma theory (Goffman), what remains behind (beyond) the masks that we wear in relationships with the others? In other words, can the existence of an authentic identity be sustained? A possible answer was found by Weber when he announced the difficulties of the self-definition of the individual, but also in characterising others. The German theorist speaks of a critical phase of the modern society—the *defensive* identifications of the "communitary" type block the evolution of *constructive*, yet uncertain identifications of the "societal" type. In other words, to categorize yourself within the boundaries of a community is a step back, a defence strategy (like an excuse, a personal limiting), while the bold identification brings prestige to the one who announces *themselves* in a way, then finding that there are others like them.

We also bring into discussion current visions on the issue of identity, following Wieseltier. The American philosopher-journalist believes that "only [they] who have an identity can understand why you want to get rid of it," in a present in which (at least in the USA) you feel suffocated by identity, not only of others but your own, because it is composed of an "overlap of irreducible entities." The danger of superposing the incomparable characteristics consists in ignoring the multiple identities to the extent that, self-sufficiently, it ignores the identity of others. Perpetually oscillating between what we are and what we would want to be, we can treat identity as the saving solution to the problem of individuality, because in the identity the obsessions, confusions and existential chaos of each are collected and ordered (Wieseltier 1997, 18). The author considers identity a double affirmation of the identity-itself (towards what is like you, him) and of the difference (towards what isn't like you or him). And then "What is your identity?" receives another interrogation as an answer—"Who are you like?"

We shall decide, perhaps, that identity=similarity, and from here the way to approval of democracy infiltrated through the breaches of identity is not a complicated path. Wieseltier (1997, 41) translates this democracy as: "Someone like me and different from me is already here with me." We must not believe that this democratic identity is silent, discreet; identity is public, the author says: "it's the way someone is known," because an identity kept secret, intimate, is just a strategy of survival, "the improvisation typical to the endangered minority." It is an impertinent attitude to apply criticism to those with a threatened existence; in America it is difficult to be what you are, with delicacy. These statements make Wieseltier easier to understand when he associates identity with epithets such as capricious and flexible for the sake of self-justification. Convinced that postmodernism has its source in inconsistency, the author attaches the lack of consistency to the false promise of uniqueness through identity. Identity is even an illusion for those who take diversity seriously, equating it to complexity. The simplicity of identity appears as opposite to the one before, hence: "not: My identity, but: my identities. In the plural there is more truth, and a greater appearance of decency."

But where does the formation of identity begin? Where the usefulness of the "multiple" identification ends, the replica emerges. If we attribute the meaning of diversity, or of the different, to the multiple we will agree with the conclusion: "There is no point to take pride in your difference, if the differences blind, if the others can't see" (Wieseltier 1997, 81). In other words, the social dialogue requires the acceptance from an individual of the elements that lead to identity, at the same time in which its interlocutor values components of personality that lead to differences between the two. Identity, Wieseltier says, is based on the attitude of reception, on the availability of the social significants to tolerate the similarities and differences that generate identities that are definitive, contextual, temporary.

The father of social psychology, Moscovici (2011, 232), finds an effective criterion of evaluating people's modes of perception, and also of the way in which "they judge and influence each other," in what he calls "the network of sympathies and antipathies." This idea completes the study of Walster & Abrahams (1972, 223) on the relationship between interpersonal attraction and social influence, the conclusion being predictable: "a nice person will be more effective in exercising a social influence than a less nice person."

Close to the American author, Mihăieş (1997) "ploughs" the same field of the identitary discourse, starting from the conviction that the identitary message of postmodernism is a fractured one (ill by rupture—A/N), equally closed and open. There, we face, at the end of the millennium, an individual with the identity repressed, incapable (as in the previous eras) of expansion of the ego, lacking the joy of affirmation from an overly accentuated pressure from the excess of imagination. How would they define their identity under conditions so harsh, of "a man who is through?" As a description of human individuality; in the form of a cultural process, within the limits of a technique—these are the offers made by Mihăieş (Ibid.) at the end of a double analysis of the individual and of the society in which they perform. It's a universal key to a profitable interpersonal communication, or exclusively the solution to the problem of alienation; identity is, ultimately, a choice, a consequence of the selection of criteria, "a form of self-isolation, even a 'doctrine of aversion'" (Wieseltier 1997, 16) (because it shows you who you are, but also who you can't be; in other words, it represents a summation of differences). To individualize yourself, the author states, you use identity and difference equally.

In a simplistic expression, identity is the "limitative, foolish, reckless assuming of what you are, of what you would want to be, of what you already imagine you became." In these figures proposed, perceived and lived nests the "moving statue of identity," as argued by Mihăieş (1997) through the seduction of the whole, excessive flexibility, self-justification, inconsistency, and irony. And yet, the Romanian author points out that the language of identity is linked to a *single* feature, despite the whole, understanding by this an attitude that is possessive at its height, coming from limitation and selfishness. Wieseltier (1997, 88) said: "I love him because he is mine." This is the language of identity. Properly translated, it means "I don't love him, I love myself." The metaphor of the "hairspray identity" is successful, since it explains the limit of the endurance of the tension between the whole and totality, between the sum of your characteristics in the idea of a complete being and totality as an identitary mark by highlighting a unique feature.

On what would be based the superiority of identity in the postmodern era? By no means on globalization, the inconsistency of personal experiences as particular sources of multiculturalism, even in America, where identity is not the same as diversity. Reunited individualities don't mean multiculturalism, and it is wrong to state it about multicultural society, because the individual can be multicultural, but not the social ensemble (Wieseltier 1997, 20).

Conclusions

Undoubtedly, a social necessity occurred within the inherent technological progress, and virtual communication seduces and, to some extent, convinces. Clearly, it is a trend that has caught on and "is worn." Publicly traded, repeated in many ways, bringing multiple powerful and durable relationships. Contested by some, with good reason. A genuine phenomenon.

References

Agnès, Y. (2011). *Introducere în jurnalism* [Introduction to Journalism]. Iaşi: Ed. Polirom.

Bădău, H. M. (2011). *Tehnici de comunicare în social media* [Communication Techniques in Social Media]. Iași: Polirom.

Brunner, R. (2000). *Psihanaliză şi societate postmodernă* [Psychoanalysis and Postmodern Society]. Timişoara: Amarcord.

Drăgan, I. (2007). *Comunicarea. Paradigme şi teorii I* [Communication: Paradigms and Theories 1]. Bucureşti: RAO.

Fidler, R. (2004). *Mediamorphosis. Să înţelegem noile media* [Mediamorphosis: Understanding the New Media]. Cluj-Napoca: Ideea Design & Print.

Ghiu, B. (2002). *Evul media sau omul terminal* [Middle Ages or The Terminal Man]. Cluj-Napoca: Ideea Design &Print.

Lovink, G. (2004). *Cultura digitală. Reflecţii critice* [Digital Culture: Critical Reflections]. Cluj-Napoca: Ideea Design & Print.

Manovich, L. (2001). *The Language of New Media*. Cambridge, MA: The MIT Press.

Mihăieş, M. (1997). Prefaţă [Preface]. In L. Wieseltier, *Împotriva identităţii*. Iaşi: Polirom.

Moscovici, S. (2011). *Influenţă socială şi schimbare socială* [Social Influence and Social Change]. Iaşi: Polirom.

Silver, D. (2000). Looking Backwards, Looking Forwards: Cyberculture Studies, 1990-2000. In D. Guantlett (Ed.), *Web. Studies*. London: Arnold Publishers.

Walster, E. & Abrahams, D. (1972). Interpersonal attraction and social influence. In J. T. Tedeschi (Ed.), *The Social Influence Processes*. Chicago, MA: Aldine Atherton.

Wieseltier, L. (1997). *Împotriva identităţii* [Against Identity]. Iaşi: Polirom.

PSYCHOLOGICAL ADAPTIVE MECHANISMS IN HOMELESS PEOPLE: A STUDY OF PEOPLE IN THE CARITAS FEDERATION NIGHT SHELTER, CATHOLIC DIOCESE OF TIMIŞOARA, ROMANIA

DĂNUŢ-IOAN CRAŞOVAN AND DELIA TOMICI

Introduction

This study is part of the first stage of a series aimed at identifying ways to adapt psychologically, represented by psychological defence mechanisms and coping mechanisms specific to various types of clinical and non-clinical populations, and atypical populations such as the reference population in this study—homeless people. By identifying mental defence in each clinical, non-clinical or atypical population (e.g. institutionalized elderly people, people without shelter, medical personnel in intensive care clinics [Răşcanu, Priceputu & Craşovan 2011], medical staff in oncology clinics [Craşovan & Priceputu 2010], or medical staff in HIV departments), a number of techniques may be developed in counselling and psychotherapy which can be effective and tailored to each medical condition or population, while the psychological defence mechanisms and coping mechanisms can serve as effective predictors in the evolution of human subjects both in a non-clinical and psychopathological condition (APA 2000/2003; 2013; Cramer 1991a; 1998; 2006; Blackman 2009; Ionescu, Jacquet & Lhote 2002). At the same time, these studies are consistent with the growing interest of researchers to analyze the psychological defence (Ionescu, Jacquet & Lhote 2002; Petraglia et al. 2009; Vaillant 1976; 1993a; 1993b) in different medical conditions, in psychotherapy, psychological counselling and other fields such as medication of mental illness, occupational selection, prevention and health education (Ionescu, Jacquet & Lhote 2002).

Accordingly, in recent years the interest of researchers with different theoretical orientations has greatly increased in analyzing psychological defence and coping mechanisms both in personality assessment (Cramer 1991a; 1991b; 1998 2006) and in psychopathology, in monitoring the defensive way of functioning, analyzing the psychological defence becoming a good tool in assessing progress and outcomes of treatment (Bond 2004). By introducing, in the latest edition of D.S.M. IV-R, a tool for analyzing psychological defence—a Scale of Defence Functioning (APA 2000/2003)—it has been recognized that the approach of the psychopathological fact is impossible without mental defence analysis.

In a series of researches on non-clinical samples from the general population (Bullitt & Farber 2002), the results do not show individual differences in the general level of maturity of defences, but demonstrate different defensive sets specific to the two types (Cramer 1991b; Watson & Sinha 1998), explained by different social arrangements that favour the emergence and development of some defences and the absence/inhibition or low functioning of other defences (Petraglia et al. 2009).

In this context this research identifies the psychological defence and coping mechanisms specific to the homeless population, techniques in psychological counselling and even psychotherapeutic intervention for beneficiaries of the Night Shelter, Father Jordan House of Caritas Federation, Catholic Diocese Timisoara, Romania and that can be adapted and made efficient for the homeless population in general.

Related to this context the following two objectives were proposed in relation to the exploratory nature of the study: to identify specific coping mechanisms in homeless people, and to identify specific psychological defence mechanisms in homeless people.

Method

Participants

The sample used includes 101 participants (N=101), namely 51 homeless people (M_{age}=46.18, SD_{age}=13.88, 14 of which were women), all beneficiaries of the services provided by the Night Shelter, Pater Jordan House of Caritas Federation, Catholic Diocese Timişoara, România, and 50 participants in the general population group (M_{age}=29.40, SD_{age}=8.72, including 21 women), assessed from March to June 2013. The development of the study assumed the administration of a Demographic Questionnaire, the DSQ 60 Questionnaire (Thygesen et al. 2008), and the COPE Questionnaire (Carver, Scheier & Weintraub 1989) on 101 subjects.

Instruments and Procedure

The Demographic questionnaire was used for the recording of demographic data and details of the participants in the research.

The **Defence Style Questionnaire 60 (DSQ 60)** was drafted by Thygesen et al. (2008). (The DSQ 60 Questionnaire Romanian version was validated in Romania on a general sample N=1011 subjects by Craşovan & Maricuţoiu [2012]). The DSQ 60 is a self-report measure with 60 items, used for the assessment of psychological defence mechanisms. The DSQ 60 scales address each of the 30 individual defence mechanisms of the DSM IV (APA 2000/2003). The score for each defence mechanism is obtained by adding the answer (chosen by the participant from a scale from 1 to 9) from the 2 items corresponding to the particular defence mechanism. The evaluation of the global defensive functioning implies computing a general score for the answers to all DSQ 60 items. This score represents a measure of the general maturity of the defensive functioning, with the high scores indicating a pronounced defensive functioning (Trijsburg et al. 2003). Thygesen et al. (2008) suggested the evaluation of the defensive style starting from the subject's answers of the DSQ-60. This perspective clearly distinguishes three levels of defence which correspond to the three levels of maturity for the defensive functioning. For each level, scores are computed through aggregation of the items that belong to each factor (Thygesen et al. 2008). A hierarchy with 7 levels of defence mechanisms (Perry 1990) was proposed as an alternative to the DSQ 60's scoring system. Similar to the maturity of the defensive functioning perspective, this alternative classifies the defence mechanisms starting from their content.

The internal consistency of the 30 scales for the DSQ 60 Romanian version is very low, with values ranging from .10 (for repression) and .77 (for retraction), with a medium value of .38 (Crașovan & Maricuțoiu 2012).

The **COPE Questionnaire** is a self-reporting instrument used for the evaluation of coping strategies elaborated by Carver, Scheier & Weintraub (1989). The Romanian version was validated for a general sample N=1009 subjects (Crașovan & Sava 2013). The Questionnaire has 60 items, and each of the 15 coping strategies is evaluated through 4 items. The rating is achieved by summing the scores from each of the 4 items corresponding to each of the 15 coping mechanisms. For example, for the positive interpretation and increase of coping mechanisms, responses are summed up to items 1, 29, 38, 59 that match this coping mechanism. The items have been used in at least three formats. One is a "dispositional" or trait-like version in which respondents report the extent to which they usually do the things listed when they are stressed. A second is a time-limited version in which respondents indicate the degree to which they actually did have each response during a particular period in the past. The third is a time-limited version in which respondents indicate the degree to which they have had each response during a period up to the present. The formats differ in their verb forms—the dispositional format is present tense, the situational-past format is past tense, and the third format is present tense progressive (I am …) or present perfect (I have been …). Regarding the psychometric properties of the original version, the Alfa Cronbach Coefficient for the 15 scales is situated between .21 (mental deactivation) and .93. The average value of the alpha coefficient for the 15 subscale is .74. For the Romanian version of COPE Questionnaire alfa Cronbach coefficient ranges from an unsatisfactory value of .48 (restraint) to an excellent value of .92 (substance consumption) and the average value of the alpha coefficient for the 15 subscales is .70 (Craşovan & Sava 2013).

As for the administration procedure, the participants were informed of the purpose of the research and their informed consent was requested, while the following questionnaires were subsequently applied in the presence of a research assistant: Demographic Questionnaire, DSQ 60 (Craşovan & Maricuţoiu 2012) and COPE Questionnaire (Craşovan & Sava 2013).

Data analysis was run using the "t" independent test under the statistic program of data analysis SPSS version 16 (Howitt & Cramer 2010) and PowerStaTim 1.0 (Sava & Maricuţoiu 2007). In this research, PowerStaTim 1.0 was used to calculate the effect size and statistical power.

Results

The results obtained are shown in Tables 2-3 and 2-4 below.

Table 2-3. Mean, standard deviation, "t" test, degrees of freedom, and probability for the coping mechanisms (N=101)

coping mechanisms	homeless people N=51		general population N=50		t	df	p
	M	SD	M	SD			
Positive reinterpretation and growth	12.20	2.62	13.14	1.86			
Mental disengagement	9.31	2.44	9.42	2.31			
Focus on and venting of emotions	10.14	3.16	10.02	2.22			
Use of instrumental social support	10.75	3.68	13.02	2.50			
Active coping	12.92	2.91	12.64	2.22			
Denial	*9.45*	*2.52*	*6.64*	*2.16*	*6.003*	*99*	*.00*
Religious coping	12.84	3.67	12.86	3.83			
Humour	6.84	3.30	9.20	3.64			
Behavioural disengagement	*9.55*	*3.07*	*7.02*	*2.00*	*4.906*	*99*	*.00*
Restraint	10.75	2.61	10.86	2.52			
Use of emotional social support	10.51	3.82	12.68	2.77			
Substance use	*6.02*	*3.26*	*4.30*	*.931*	*3.614*	*99*	*.00*
Acceptance	11.33	3.09	11.38	2.42			
Suppression of competing activities	11.45	3.03	11.32	2.34			
Planning	12.49	2.95	13.26	2.37			

Discussion and Conclusions

In this case, for the first objective of the study, as can be seen from the data presented in Table 2-3 above, statistical analysis revealed significant differences between the homeless people and general population groups following 3 coping mechanisms of the 15 operationalized with COPE: denial, behavioural disengagement and substance use.

Substance use as a coping mechanism specific to the homeless population has also been reported by Gelberg, Andersen & Leake (2000).

Analyzing the coping mechanisms predominantly used by homeless participants, the existence of ineffective coping strategies, predominantly avoidant, can be observed

In terms of the size of the effect, the existence of medium to high effect size value (d_{denial}=1.20, $d_{behavioral\ disengagement}$=.98, $d_{substance\ use}$=.72) for all coping mechanisms identified as specific for homeless people can be identified at the same time as the existence of a high statistical power (st $power_{denial}$=1, st $power_{behavioral\ disengagement}$=.98, st $power_{substance\ use}$=.83), taking as reference values given by Popa (2008), Sava (2011) and Sava & Maricuţoiu (2007).

Table 2-4. Mean, standard deviation, "t" test, degrees of freedom and probability for the psychological defence mechanisms (N=101)

Psychological defence mechanisms	homeless people		general population		t	df	p
	N=51		N=50				
	M	SD	M	SD			
altruism	14.88	4.02	15.00	2.78			
passive-aggressive	7.57	4.30	6.12	4.13			
suppression	11.45	4.33	11.50	3.61			
sublimation	11.08	4.64	11.32	4.48			
splitting/other	*11.37*	*4.38*	*9.02*	*4.59*	*2.633*	*99*	*.01*
rationalization	12.57	3.96	11.56	3.67			
humour	8.18	4.77	11.06	4.12			
projection	*11.67*	*4.99*	*6.06*	*3.22*	*6.713*	*99*	*.00*
reaction formation	11.61	4.53	11.02	3.51			
self-observation	13.55	4.28	13.62	3.31			
denial	*10.39*	*4.22*	*7.50*	*3.54*	*3.723*	*99*	*.00*
devaluation of other	8.96	4.69	8.00	4.17			
projective identification	9.86	4.62	9.58	4.28			
dissociation	*9.90*	*5.28*	*7.42*	*3.97*	*2.670*	*99*	*.00*
self-assertion	13.35	4.04	13.32	3.73			
omnipotence	8.24	4.79	7.80	4.46			
acting-out	8.76	5.43	10.00	4.41			
devaluation/self	7.47	4.41	6.48	4.00			
fantasy	*8.16*	*5.67*	*5.58*	*3.60*	*2.731*	*99*	*.00*
withdrawal	*13.53*	*5.34*	*10.74*	*4.49*	*2.835*	*99*	*.00*
intellectualization	*11.10*	*4.48*	*8.00*	*3.87*	*3.715*	*99*	*.00*
splitting/self	*9.41*	*5.48*	*6.70*	*4.14*	*2.805*	*99*	*.00*
displacement	8.67	3.84	9.12	4.12			
repression	10.00	5.15	8.50	3.55			
idealization	10.78	5.34	10.14	4.86			
isolation	*11.00*	*4.20*	*7.98*	*4.45*	*3.504*	*99*	*.00*
help-rejecting complaining	*9.61*	*4.62*	*6.28*	*3.61*	*4.023*	*99*	*.00*
undoing	10.45	4.66	8.86	3.91			
anticipation	12.96	4.29	12.20	3.35			
affiliation	11.16	5.82	12.10	3.97			

Regarding the second objective of the study, namely to identify psychological defence mechanisms used by homeless people, as can be seen from the data presented in Table 2-4 above, statistical analysis identified statistically significant effects between the homeless people and general population groups following 10 psychological defence mechanisms of the 30 psychological defence mechanisms operationalized with DSQ 60, and taken into consideration: splitting/other, projection, denial, dissociation, fantasy, withdrawal, intellectualization, splitting/self, isolation and help-rejecting complaining.

In the case of psychological defence mechanisms the use of the four mechanisms listed in the Affective Adjustment Style (dissociation, fantasy, intellectualization and isolation [see Craşovan & Maricuţoiu 2012]) can be observed, along with the use of four of the five psychological defence mechanisms of the Defensive Style (splitting/other, projection, splitting/self and help-rejecting complaining [see Craşovan & Maricuţoiu 2012]), mechanisms which with denial and withdrawal show a low or even ineffective level of defence.

In this case, the indicators of effect size and statistical power for the 10 psychological defence mechanisms identified as specific to homeless people have shown values of the effect size from medium to optimal levels ($d_{splitting/other=}$.52, d_{denial}=.74, $d_{dissociation}$=.53, $d_{fantasy}$=.54, $d_{withdrawal}$=.57, $d_{intellectualization}$=.74, $d_{splitting/self}$=.56, $d_{isolation=}$.70 and $d_{help\text{-}rejecting\ complaining}$=.81), and even high in the case of projection ($d_{projection}$=1.34), and in the case of statistical power the existence of values from medium to optimal (st $power_{splitting/other}$=.51, st $power_{projection}$=.1, st $power_{denial}$=.86, st $power_{dissociation}$=.52, st $power_{fantasy}$=.55, st $power_{withdrawal}$=.59, st $power_{intellectualization}$=.86, st $power_{splitting/self}$=.58, st $power_{isolation}$=.82 and st $power_{help\text{-}rejecting\ complaining}$=.91), taking as reference values given by Popa (2008), Sava (2011) and Sava & Maricuţoiu (2007).

In conclusion, as specific to homeless people the study shows the coping mechanisms of denial, behavioural disengagement and substance use, and the psychological defence mechanisms of splitting/other, projection, denial, dissociation, fantasy, withdrawal, intellectualization, splitting/self, isolation and help-rejecting complaining.

Overall, the ways to adapt psychologically for the participants who are homeless indicate an inefficient adaptation of the low level.

Based on these results, psychological counselling or psychotherapeutic intervention techniques will seek ways of improving psychological adjustment by replacing the psychological defence and coping mechanisms used by homeless participants that are immature and ineffective with effective defence and coping mechanisms with a high level of adaptation.

References

American Psychiatric Association. (2013). *Diagnostic and Statistical Manual of Mental Disorders*. Washington, DC: American Psychiatric Association.

—. (2000). *Diagnostic and Statistical Manual of Mental Disorders*. Washington, DC: American Psychiatric Association.

—. (2003). *Manual de Diagnostic și Statistică a Tulburărilor Mentale (DSM-IV-TR)* [Diagnostic and Statistical Manual of Mental Disorders (DSM-IV-TR)]. București: Editura Asociației Psihiatrilor Liberi din România.

Blackman, J. S. (2009). *101 apărări. Cum se autoprotejează mintea* [101 defenses. How the mind defends itself]. București: Trei.

Bullitt, C. W. & Farber B. A. (2002). Gender differences in defensive style. *Journal of the American Academy of Psychoanalysis 30*: 35-51.

Carver, C. S., Scheier, M. F. & Weintraub, J. K. (1989). Assessing coping strategies: A theoretically based approach. *Journal of Personality and Social Psychology 56*: 267-283.

Cramer, P. (1991a). Development of defense mechanisms: *Theory, research, and assessment*. New York, NY: Springer-Verlag.

—. (1991b). Anger and the use of defense mechanismsin college students. *Journal of Personality 59 (1)*: 39-55.

—. (1998). Coping and Defense Mechanisms: What's the Difference? *Journal of Personality 66*: 919-946.

—. (2006). *Protecting the self: Defense mechanisms in action*. New York, NY: The Guilford Press.

Crașovan, D. I. & Priceputu, M. (2010). Exploratory study on coping and defense mechanisms of medical staff in medical clinics (oncology) with patients in terminal stages of disease. *Health in context: 24th Annual Conference of the European Health Psychology Society, Cluj-Napoca, Romania.*

Crașovan, D. I. & Maricuțoiu, L.P. (2012). Adaptation of the Defensive Style Questionnaire 60 (DSQ-60) within a Romanian sample. *Cognition, Brain, Behavior. An Interdisciplinary Journal 16*: 509-528. Online:http://www.cbbjournal.ro/index.php?option=com_content&task=view&id=509&Itemid=59.

Crașovan, D. I. & Sava, A. F. (2013). Translation, adaptation and validation on Romanian population of COPE Questionnaire for coping mechanisms analysis. *Cognition, Brain, Behavior. An Interdisciplinary Journal* XVII (1): 61-76. Online: http://www.cbbjournal.ro/index.php?option=com_content&task=view&id=515&Itemid=60.

Gelberg, L., Andersen, R. M. & Leake, B. D. (2000). The Behavioral Model for Vulnerable Populations: application to medical care use and outcomes for homeless people. *Health services research 34* (6): 1273.

Howitt, D. & Cramer, H. (2010). *Introducere în SPSS pentru psihologie* [Introduction to SPSS for Psychology]. Iaşi: Polirom.

Ionescu, Ş., Jacquet, C.-L. & Lhote, C. (2002). *Mecanismele de apărare. Teorie şi aspecte clinice* [Defense mechanisms: Theory and clinical aspects]. Iaşi: Polirom.

Perry, J. C. (1990). *Defense Mechanism Rating Scales*. Boston, MA: Harvard Medical School.

Petraglia, J., Thygesen, K. L., Lecours, S. & Drapeau, M. (2009). Gender differences in self-reported defense mechanisms: A study using the new Defense Style Questionnaire-60. *American Journal of Psychotherapy 63*: 87-99.

Popa, M. (2008). *Statistică pentru psihologie. Teorie şi aplicaţii SPSS* [Statistics for Psychology: SPSS Theory and Applications]. Iaşi: Polirom.

Răşcanu, R., Priceputu, M. & Craşovan, D. I. (2011). The analysis of defense mechanisms and coping strategies in the medical personnel of the intensive care ward, University hospital Timisoara. *International Conference of Integrative Psychotherapy "Approaching well-being from an integrative and interdisciplinary perspective," Bucharest, Romania.*

Sava, F. & Maricuţoiu, L.-P. (2007). *PowerStaTim. Manualul utilizatorului* [PowerStaTim. User's Manual]. Timişoara: Editura Universităţii de Vest.

Sava, F. A. (2011). *Analiza datelor în cercetarea psihologica* [Data Analysis in Psychological Research]. Cluj-Napoca: ASCR.

Thygesen, K. L., Drapeau, M., Trijsburg, R. W., Lecours, S. & de Roten, Y. (2008). Assessing defence styles: Factor structure and psychometric properties of the new Defence Style Questionnaire 60 (DSQ-60). *The International Journal of Psychology and Psychological Therapy 8*: 171-181.

Trijsburg, R. W., Bond, M., Drapeau, M., Thygesen, K. L., de Roten, Y. & Duivenvoorden, H. J. (2003). *Defense Style Questionnaire 60: Development and psychometric evaluation*. Paper presented at the University of Lausanne, Switzerland.

Vaillant, G. E. (1976). Natural history of male psychological health: The relation of choice of ego mechanism of defense to adult ajustement *Archives of General Psychiatry* 33: 535-545.

—. (1993a). *Wisdom of the ego: Sources of resilience in adult life*. Cambridge: HUP.

—. (1993b). *The wisdom of the ego*. Cambridge: HUP.

Watson, D. C. & Sinha, B. K. (1998). Gender, age, and cultural differences in the defense style questionnaire-40. *Journal of Clinical Psychology 54*: 67-75.

MULTIPLE INTELLIGENCES FOR BETTER INCLUSION

MARIA CONSTANTINESCU
AND CORNEL CONSTANTINESCU

Introduction

This study aims to develop a learning resource for specialists in the field of social work and adult education working with people with no qualifications or who are low skilled. At its base sits the Multiple Intelligences Theory (MI) developed by Howard Gardner (1999), whose *Frames of Mind* (1983) had a great impact and was a manifesto against IQ. He challenged the psychometric-standard approach (Terman 1925; Spearman 1927) based on intelligence tests (Binet & Simon 1905) that consider intelligence as a general cognitive factor, arguing that there is no single monolithic type of intelligence that underpins success in life, but a wide range of intelligence for new possibilities. His approach to researching the traditional images of intelligence finished by creating different profiles and proposing the idea of a single intelligence factor "S," where S means specific.

The basic idea of our project is removing the transmission pattern of poverty and exclusion from one generation to another by training the marginalized and disadvantaged citizens regarding their ability to more easily solve everyday problems in different areas, without being kept apart due to their area of origin. The whole experience of the individual from a socially disadvantaged family produces a habitus less developed, used by the individual in future experiences. Lack of education and training will become a habit for them in living and acting according to the norms and values developed. In our study, our preoccupation is the "traditional vulnerability," in which "the individual acts in virtue of habit or state of social passivity which is transmitted due to the influence of the environment" (Vladu 2010, 39). The case of the beneficiaries from socially disadvantaged families is that they are disadvantaged, which is transmitted from one generation to another. Using multiple intelligence specialists in social work and adult education can provide help to socially disadvantaged citizens and those at risk of social exclusion, providing them with innovative learning environments, facilitating learning and improving skills in the following areas: abilities for "learning to learn" skills of financial management, parenting skills, employability skills and entrepreneurship.

The point of view that shows the many facets of intelligence (Thurstone 1960; Wechsler 1967; Guilford 1967; Gardner 1993; Goleman 2005) provides a broader image of the human being and the ability or potential for success than the IQ standard. The operative word in the MI model of Gardner is multiple, and his model goes far beyond the standard concept of IQ as a singular and invariable factor. In terms of everyday life, all intelligences act in an individual, specific harmony. Gardner (1999) defines intelligence as "a psychobiological potential to process information that can be activated in a cultural setting to solve problems or create products that are of value in a culture."

The author of MI theory discusses nine intelligences that are relatively autonomous (howardgardner.com). His list includes, in the first instance, the two types of standard intelligence: learning, verbal intelligence (IL) and logical-mathematical intelligence (LMI). He also includes the spatial capacity (IS), bodily-kinaesthetic intelligence (ICC), and musical intelligence (MI), involving the sense of rhythm and sounds and facilitating composition. To all this he adds the personal intelligences (IP), which can be interpersonal capacities (interpersonal intelligence) that make people able to recognize and make differences between feelings and intentions, and intrapsychic capacities (intrapersonal intelligence) which helps them to understand to lead their own lives.

Gardner and other researchers have left a vast ocean of emotions unexplored that makes inner life and relationships so complex, compelling and often confused. Goleman (2001), with John D. Mayer and Peter Salovey (1997) as precursors, provides an expanded proposal of a model of what it means to be smart, and puts emotions as central skills needed for life. Goleman believes that there is intelligence in emotions, and that emotions can influence intelligence (Constantinescu 2004, 163).

In his list, Gardner included two other types of intelligence, namely naturalistic intelligence (IN) and existential intelligence (EI). Human beings possess all nine in varying degrees, but each individual has a different intelligence profile. These intelligences demonstrate that education could be improved by evaluating intelligence profiles of the trainees in order to design training activities according to these needs.

Methods and Techniques

Using the key points of the Multiple Intelligences Theory has developed a set of tools, examples, strategies and best practices for teachers of adults and social professionals to facilitate their work with socially disadvantaged groups. Evaluation and validation were tested by organizing national workshops and key activities of the project in four target countries (Portugal, Spain, Romania and Germany), partners in the project. Countries that have implemented workshops were selected based on their socio-economic context. Thus, Portugal, Spain and Romania have major problems with those who leave school early and have a very high risk of being excluded from society due to the low level of skills in many of the key areas of competence. These people lack the skills required for the labour market, and therefore it is important to allocate resources to address this problem. Workshops were implemented in January and February 2013 with an aim to test and validate the pilot version of the Manual "New ways, easy answers to difficult problems," and to specifically evaluate the techniques and methods to be more effective and useful for adult trainers and health professional social workers with disadvantaged people. In this way, this leads to promoting the development of financial management skills, active skills for employment and entrepreneurship, parenting skills and the ability to learn, using information from the multiple intelligence theory.

The workshops had a common structure, coordinated and facilitated by a facilitator, two experts in the field, all with experience in providing training, knowledge and experience in the MI theory of dynamic groups. In Romania over 150 people have been contacted through e-mail and telephone. By e-mail associations and foundations in the target group (over 110) were contacted, and by telephone and e-mail previously surveyed respondents were informed in order to achieve the needs analysis. Data gathered during the workshop on February 6 and 7, 2013 were established by agreement with the people willing to participate in this activity, lasting for sixteen hours over two days.

Workshop Participants Attending the workshop were 26 professionals from the socio-educational field; 93% graduates with university degrees and 7% with professional training.

Years of Experience (average): four months to seventeen years.

Professional Background: teacher in special education, psychologist teacher, school counsellor, social worker, coordinator of school mediators, school mediator, school assessor for the children with SEN, adult trainer specializing in inclusive policy and practice, teacher psychopedagogue, school social worker in special education, assistant for young people infected with HIV.

Tools for collecting feedback from the target group and experts. Feedback from participants was collected using a questionnaire (with a scale of 1 to 5, where 1 represents the level "excellent" and 5 represents the level "inappropriately," using the Lickert model) and oral feedback. The following instruments to evaluate the testing and validation were proposed: a specific questionnaire to collect feedback from the workshop facilitator and other experts focused more on qualitative than quantitative; a specific questionnaire to collect feedback from workshop participants regarding the effectiveness of implemented techniques (validation) and their satisfaction of the organization of the workshop, facilities and location; manual content, teaching approaches and suggestions from workshop subsequent events; organizing a **focus group** workshop during implementation in order to discuss and exchange views on this subject; **face to face interviews to assess the follow-up activities**, putting into practice the knowledge gained during the workshop. Between two and five interviews of the workshop participants are conducted. The purpose of the interviews is to assess the impact of the manual in the professional life of the participants. It is also interesting to see if the training implemented in the workshop had a multiplying effect (of the transfer of knowledge from the other fellow workshop participants, contacts, etc.).

Results and Discussion

The participants in the workshop received information about the project and its objectives, teaching materials (pilot version of the Manual "New ways, easy answers to difficult problems") and objectives of the test phase. Also, the basics in terms of social inclusion using MI theory to make learning more appropriate, attractive and light, enhancing the motivation of instructors, were explained to the participants. All parts of the manual were tested, i.e. good practices, theoretical approaches and practical activities. Students worked some exercises on how to recognize and use various intelligences identified by Gardner. The manual includes different types of activities assuming three different levels of knowledge and skills in the management of MI theory and exercises were grouped into three levels: basic, intermediate and advanced, depending on the knowledge of the beneficiaries. Seventeen examples have been practicing the four categories of skills that promote social inclusion by increasing employability (4), to facilitate the management of financial and management mistakes to avoid risk and borrowing (2), to encourage better parenting behaviours (5) and involvement in trust for new learning opportunitics (6). The four skill areas were chosen because of their major role in promoting inclusion understood as developing an employment policies workforce contributing to the social and professional integration of vulnerable groups.

> Active inclusion aims to ensure non-discriminatory access to the labour market and improving living and working conditions by implementing integrated programs that provide sufficient income to ensure the needs of living, quality services of general interest, and labour market integration programs to the most vulnerable people. (Zamfir & Zamfir 2011, 18)

Some of the exercises were individually crafted, while others were solved in teams of four to five people. Participants have gladly engaged in program activities, as the facilitator made a number of materials available (flipchart, TV and video, paper and pens, paper, etc.) and created an atmosphere of trust and working.

Feedback from the students was positive (the mean score ranged between 1.5 and 2.5) in terms of satisfaction with the workshop organization, location, facilities, activities and pedagogical approach developed. All participants received a certificate of participation and considered granting a certificate for professional development. Most people surveyed responded affirmatively on using these techniques in their work. Among the reasons cited were: it is an important resource of practical exercises to stimulate different types of intelligence, it improves teaching, vocational training and personal development, and it informs the theory of multiple intelligences. Favourable scores (2.5) were obtained for the sections Good Practice and how to apply MI theory in Social Work, and How to Build a Profile of Social Intelligence, the middle score obtained was not positive, and almost all participants found it difficult to elaborate a social intelligence profile. In addition, regarding the section "How to use the Manual," the participants expressed their disagreement with the content quality, of which some aspects are not clear, easy to understand or reliable, especially regarding the advanced level of competence. At the basic level, they understood the need to know the principles and basic concepts of the MI theory and realized that there are different intelligences. What MI theory can provide at this level is a more extensive view of the skills that people possess. At the intermediate level, the difference lies in how they can apply MI theory in an educational context, and use all types of intelligences for people who have trained. At the advanced level, you can work to balance individual profiles, recognizing the particular type of abilities in each client, etc. This level is more complex and informed, with participants proposing to deepen the involvement of other courses. In this sense, their feedback was positive, with three quarters of the students expressing their consent to participate in a course in the UK International Grundvig on the basis of the pilot manual.

Expectations regarding the workshop: Identifying ways of helping disadvantaged youth and/or marginalized people to integrate more easily into society, acquire knowledge and develop skills to improve business counselling and the provision of working tools or guidelines that can be used in professional and personal life, etc.

Feedback from face to face interviews to assess follow-up activities: the practical implementation of knowledge gained from the workshop was a positive one, because three of the five surveyed said they have used this knowledge in their courses (with students of social and educational sciences) and were disseminated among colleagues, considering that MI theory can make learning more appropriate, more attractive and easier for trainers of adults and social professionals, facilitating their work with socially disadvantaged groups, the workshop participants with other colleagues, contacts, etc.

Conclusions

Smart ways for better inclusion is a project intended to break the pattern of poverty, social exclusion and its transfer from one generation to another by empowering marginalized and disadvantaged citizens to easily manage daily problems in various areas.

In social practice, social service beneficiaries from disadvantaged families are constantly met, with disadvantage being transmitted from one generation to another. This encourages dependency on social services that appeal to those services, and has become a habit for families. Social workers and adult education instructors are constantly faced with such challenges, and they need many different people with knowledge of daily problems to solve them. Adopting MI theory as a framework for their work, social workers and adult educators will better understand human behaviour, with pluralistic access to their basic skills. This means that MI theory can be considered a tool for improving the skills of specialists in adult education and social assistance (target group) when working with disadvantaged citizens living in disadvantaged communities (beneficiaries) and to better understand the full range of the important skills knowledge of the individual.

In addition, MI theory can provide a closer look at the skills that people possess. In this way, the opportunity to meet and solve the challenges is broad, decreasing the dependence on others and social services, and there is the opportunity to observe the behaviour and identify different types of skills that people who are trained have, useful in helping their work either through a recovery plan or in preparation.

The project aims to develop a set of tools (a manual and a training course) with innovative approaches to adult trainers and specialists in the field of social assistance to promote adaptation of their teaching techniques and learning to different styles and profiles of intelligence of disadvantaged and marginalized citizens involved in training contexts.

Acknowledgement

This study is part of the project INPATH (www.spi.pt/inpath) in which I participated as a member of the project team. Thanks to Associate Professor Georgeta Chirlesan, the project coordinator and the entire team.

References

—. *INPATH*. Online: www.spi.pt/inpath

Binet, A. & Simon, Th. (1905). Binet Simon Intelligence Test. *L'Année Psychologique 12*: 191-244..

Constantinescu, M. (2004). *Competenţa socială şi competenţa profesională* [Social Competence and Professional Competence]. Bucureşti: Editura Economică

Gardner, H. (1993). *Frames of Mind: The Theory of Multiple Intelligences.* New York, NY: Basic Books.

Gardner, H. *Howard Gardner*. Online: http://howardgardner.com/

Gardner, H. (1999). *Intelligence reframed. Multiple intelligences for the 21st century*. New York, NY: Basic Books.

Goleman, D. (2001). *Emotional Intelligence. Why It Can Matter More Than I.Q.* New York, NY: Bantam Books.

Guilford, J. P. (1967). *The Nature of Human Inteligence*. New York, NY: McGraw-Hill.

Spearman, Ch. (1927). *The Abilities of Man*. Londra: Macmillan.

Terman, L. M. (1925). *Genetic studies of genius. Mental and physical traits of a thousand gifted children 1.* Stanford, CA: Stanford University Press.

Thurstone, L. L. (1960). The Measurement of Values. Chicago, IL: I.U.

Vladu, V. (Ed.). (2010). *Manual de bune practici sociale* [A Handbook of Good Social Practices]. Cluj-Napoca: Risoprint.

Wechsler, D. (1967). *La mesure de l'intelligence de l'adulte* [The Measure of Adult's Intelligence]. Paris: PUF.

Zamfir, C. & Zamfir, E. (Eds.). (2011). *Raport de cercetare privind economia socială in Romania din perspectivă europeană comparată* [Research Report on Social Economics in Romania from a Compared European Perspective]. Bucureşti.

ALTRUISM AND INDIVIDUALISM IN FUTURE SOCIAL WORKERS

DAN-IOAN DASCĂLU

Introduction

As we speak, fierce debates are taking place worldwide, discussing the social assistance system, the possibilities of its reform and efficiency, and the best ways of professional training for those who will work in this system. Obviously, such debates cannot bypass the issue of values underpinning social work and the motivations of those working in this field. With the changes at the societal level, other changes occur in the values underlying the social assistance system and social workers' motivations. This problem arising in our country leads to, on the one hand, the profound political, economic, social, and cultural changes that occurred after 1990, and on the other a certain amount of confusion about the value system inherent in such profound changes.

We wish to bring to attention several views on the relationship between altruism and individualism as values cherished by those preparing for the social work profession. These views are based on actual research conducted at the "Stefan cel Mare" University of Suceava in 2013 on students of the social work study program. The first research question was to establish the place altruism occupies among the motivations of those who choose the social work profession. Secondly, we were interested in targeting students in terms of their organizational culture along the individualism-collectivism axis, and thirdly, we wanted to see whether there is an association between altruistic motivational orientations and location on the individualism-collectivism axis.

However, before presenting our research methodology, results and conclusions, we believe it is necessary to offer a few introductory explanations of the concepts of individualism and altruism.

In the late twentieth and early twenty-fist centuries, we can talk about a revival of individualism worldwide. Some call it the "second individualistic revolution" (Lipovetsky 1983, 19); a new individualism, with a system of values and behaviour patterns slightly different from those of the early modern era. Such remodelling and expansion of individualism were brought about by a number of processes such as globalization, the planetary imposition of consumerism and affirmation of the knowledge society, and the fall of communism in Eastern Europe. The debates on individualism have a fairly long history. Modernity has established individualism as an ideology, the foundation of economic and political thought. It is linked politically to the capitalist market economy and democracy. Modern theories of democracy award the individual and their interests in the central role in the political system. From this perspective, individualism is related to ensuring political participation and the observation of human rights.

Although the twentieth century has been largely dominated by collectivist ideologies, especially the totalitarian left or right, which resulted in some reduction of the interest in individualism, we can notice, especially after the failure of totalitarianism systems, a resurgence in the concern for modern forms of individualism. The "personalization process" (Lipovetsky 1983, 10) argues that it is characteristic of contemporary individualism, which requires, at societal level, the minimum possible for individual constraints and, at the same time, the ensuring of as many choices, together with as little coercion, as possible and potentially boundless understanding. Personalization "promotes and embodies a fundamental value, that of personal fulfillment, of respect for subjective singularity and incomparable personality, whatever the forms of control and homogenization" (Ibid., 13). Seen from this perspective, individualism is again related to humanism: "Sharing the model of an emancipated individual, individualism is a brand of humanism, drawing an ideal world in which every human being can develop and become itself" (Singly 2005, 10).

Discussions on individualism require us to consider a broad definition for this concept, for example the one proposed by Dumont: "We designate individualistic, as opposed to holism, an ideology that values the individual and neglects or subordinates the social whole" (Dumond 1983, 304). Such a definition exempts us from a debate on the different types and forms of individualism that have no place here. It is necessary to note, however, that we use the term individualism in our research in the sense given by Geert Hofstede (2001, 209), who spoke of a dimension of organizational culture: individualism-collectivism, alluding to some extent to the distinction made known by F. Tönnies between community and society: "Individualism is characteristic of societies in which ties between individuals are weak: they expect everyone to care for themselves and their close family." By contrast: "collectivism characterizes societies in which people are integrated from birth into strong internal groups, closely united, which continue throughout their life to protect them in exchange for unquestioning loyalty" (Hofstede, Hofstede & Minkov 2012, 96). Viewed from this perspective, as a dimension of organizational culture, individualism does not seem to oppose altruism. We must, however, make some remarks on this issue.

The opposition between altruism and individualism, specific primarily to common knowledge, is based on an improper interpretation of individualism which considers it identical to selfishness. If we consider altruism as "that which is opposed to selfishness, that is, the willingness to do good to others, without taking into account a consciously planned and intentional self-interest" (Wosińska 2005, 255), then obviously it opposes individualism seen as selfishness. This made, for instance, S. Moscovici (1998, 62) state that: "the problem of altruism has been posed keenly in our Western society based on the priority of interest and the individual." The dispute dates back to the second half of the nineteenth century, and had H. Spencer and E. Durkheim as its main exponents. Spencer had taken individualism to the limit of social selfishness. Rightly criticizing such a position, Durkheim (1987, 16) would redraw the humanistic milestones of individualism, arguing that it: "is not glorification of the self, but of the individual in general. It is triggered not by selfishness but by sympathy for all that is human, a deep compassion for all the pain and human miseries, a more ardent need to combat and soften them, and a greater thirst for justice."

Moreover, a series of experimental social psychology researches has shown that "willingness to help a stranger ranks higher in individualistic cultures than in collectivistic ones" (Wosińska 2005, 258).

The values of individualism do not contradict the practice of social work. Rather, they actually occupy a prominent place among the overall values of a social worker. If "faith in the uniqueness and dignity of every person and faith in the client's right to self-determination" are core values in social work premises (Alexiu 2011, 536), they are also the values of individualism.

What we were particularly interested in during our research was the possibility to associate the individualistic dimension of organizational culture with the altruistic motivations for choosing a career as a social worker.

Research Methodology

The research was conducted in May 2013 at the Stefan cel Mare University of Suceava. The subjects of the research were students of the Social Work undergraduate program in the first to third years of study. There were 143 students involved, representing almost all the students enrolled in this program. In terms of the structure of the group of subjects, the majority were female (92%) and aged between 18 and 25 (87%). The method used in the research was the questionnaire technique of the psycho-sociological survey. As a research tool we used a questionnaire which included a Professional Values Inventory and an instrument proposed and used by Hofstede in his research on organizational culture, Values Survey Module 1994.

The inventory of professional values, proposed by D. E. Super and adapted to Romania by S. Chelcea, comprises 45 items which correspond to 15 dimensions on the labour motivation scale: altruism, aesthetic, intellectual stimulation, professional success, independence, prestige, leadership, economic benefits, occupational security, physical environment, relations with superiors, relations with colleagues, lifestyle, and variety (Chelcea 1994, 102–104). Altruism means the opportunity to contribute to the good of others; aesthetic values refer to the ability to create beautiful objects and contribute to the embellishment of the world; intellectual stimulation is related to the possibility of lifelong education, of learning those professions that make autonomous reflection possible; professional success allows subjects to enjoy rewards by exercising their profession; independence occurs in those professions in which people can work according to their own planning; prestige refers to the respect of others and the social importance given to professional performance; leadership requires the ability to coordinate the work of others; the economic benefits are related to a good remuneration; occupational security requires job safety and individual security at one's workplace; the physical environment refers to the external conditions of employment; relations with superiors link to the existence of a fair boss, whom one can trust to have good relations with; relations with colleagues refer to good relations with the members of the working staff; lifestyle is linked to the ability to organize your own workplace; diversity refers to the ability to pursue a diversified activity, and creativity means the ability to do new things in one's line of work.

For each item, which presents an element of work environment or labour content, subjects are supposed to show how important they consider them on a scale of five levels: very important (5), important (4), averagely important (3), less important (2), unimportant (1). Each of the fifteen motivational dimensions above corresponds to three items. In this way it is possible to calculate the score of this dimension that can vary from 3 (unimportant) to 15 (very important).

VSM '94 includes 26 questions related to several dimensions of organizational culture. Items relating to the dimensions of organizational culture are also on a scale from 1 to 5, 1 meaning "We were interested in this research only in the size of individualism-collectivism." We calculated the rate of individualism (IDV), which has a value between 0 and 100, although in theory it could take values less than 0 or greater than 100. A value close to 100 means strong individualism, while one close to 0 means strong collectivism.

Research Results

After we processed the data, the Professional Values Inventory displayed the following average scores:

Table 2-5. Average Scores for Professional Values

Professional Values	Average	Standard Deviation
1. Physical environment	13.09	1.70
2. Relations with superiors	13.37	1.51
3. Altruism	13.32	1.76
4. Relations with colleagues	13.14	1.61
5. Lifestyle	13.13	1.88
6. Occupational security	12.84	1.97
7. Creativity	12.62	1.84
8. Professional success	12.56	1.85
9. Economic benefits	12.39	2.07
10. Prestige	11.92	1.91
11. Intellectual stimulation	11.68	1.64
12. Independence	11.66	1.96
13. Aesthetic	11.63	1.97
14. Variety	11.22	2.02
15. Leadership	9.80	2.61

It is interesting to observe the way in which these professional values associate with one another.

Table 2-6. Correlations among Professional Values

Professional Values	Altruism	Aesthetic	Intellectual stimulation	Professional success	Independence	Prestige	Leadership	Economic benefits	Occupational security	Physical environment	Relations with superiors	Relations with colleagues	Lifestyle	Variation	Creativity
3	1	.26	.18	.29	.28	.32	.26	.37	.29	.172	.23	.12	.18	.31	.32
13		1	.46	.58	.58	.407	.49	.31	.41	.49	.34	.48	.45	.56	.51
11			1	.56	.38	.38	.42	.46	.42	.43	.40	..41	.45	.48	.46
8				1	.51	.39	43	42	.61	.68	.58	.55	.60	.45	.61
12					1	.38	.61	.44	.45	.44	.46	.32	.30	.50	.37
10						1	.52	.30	.36	.41	.43	.57	59	30	36
15							1	.39	.40	.38	.44	.37	.38	.41	.39
9								1	.57	.43	.56	.35	.43	.49	.24
6									1	.71	.52	.43	.51	.38	.31
1										1	.61	.60	.64	.33	.46
2											1	.59	.68	.42	.40
4												1	.66	.38	.42
5													1	.36	.36
14														1	.41
7															1

We can notice that altruism ranks third among professional values, very close to the first two. However, examining the correlations between professional values, altruism appears in a special way. If each of the others is associated, sometimes very strongly, with others, forming genuine motivational chains, altruism is associated only weakly with only three other values. We may suspect, for example, that occupational security is associated in the minds of subjects with professional success, economic benefits, good physical working environments, and good relations with superiors or colleagues. Association coefficients (Pearson) show a significant link between these professional values. The emergence of altruism among the top professional values is quite natural, given the specific professional nature of social work. We certainly do not know whether it was this value that made the students choose their future profession, or the educational influence to which they were subjected in college that accounts for their adherence to altruism as a core professional value.

Regarding the relationship between altruism and individualism, in statistical terms we cannot talk about any association. The value of the

Pearson Association Coefficient (0.032) says it all in this regard. In fact, individuality, as measured by Hofstede, is not associated with any of the professional values in the inventory we used. It is normal, to some extent, because we deal with different things, on the one hand with values underpinning work motivation, and on the other with a certain vision about the role and functioning of organizations to which the subject belongs, including professional ones. However, we must not forget Hofstede, Hofstede & Minkov's (2012, 96–97) remark that there are significant differences in terms of work goals between the subjects oriented toward individualism and those oriented toward collectivism. Those oriented toward the individualist pole are concerned about personal time—that is to have a job that leaves plenty of time for personal life, for freedom, an exciting activity that will give them a sense of personal fulfilment. As for those oriented toward the collectivist pole, the things that become more important are the physical working conditions, the opportunities for professional training, and the fact that they can use their skills to work fully. This is a distinction mentioned before between the independence of the employee from the organization, with individualism, and their dependence on the organization, with collectivism. In our case, we can see that the professional values cherished by students are the physical environment, while values such as independence, variety and creativity are placed last. It would seem, therefore, that we are dealing with a rather collectivist orientation of students, even though such a statement may seem an exaggeration.

However, the individualism index calculated by the application of VSM '94 shows, for the subjects studied, an average value of 56.74. This is a value close to that obtained, for example, by Alin Gavreliuc on a sample representative of Banat (Gavreliuc 2011, 149–150). The value found by the Timisoara Professor was 50, placing the sample investigated on the edge between dependent collectivism and dependent individualism. Our research was not conducted on a sample representative of Bukovina, but on a group of young students with fairly high levels of education, with prospective jobs, but also with the common desire to evade the guardianship of their family and the community they belong to. This was shown by the qualitative interviews conducted after the questionnaires. Hence, probably, a higher score index in favour of individualism.

It seems that in our research we identify a certain type of individualism. As early as eight decades ago, Constantin Rădulescu-Motru (1938, 162) called it "the individualism of the Romanian soul." This individualism, the Romanian psychologist and philosopher argued, was of a different nature than the individualism of Western Europe. It was about an individualism of the soul, not an institutional individualism, which sometimes combines anarchic individual impulses with respect to the traditions of the community, and is directed against others, seen as enemies, not competitors. Based on the suggestion by Rădulescu-Motru, Alin Gavreliuc conducted field research in recent years and proposed the concept of "self-contained individualism." According to Gavreliuc (2011, 153):

> autarchic individualism involves enhancement of individual resources in self-fulfillment, but in a social context characterized by poor community solidarity (hence the qualification as autarchic), it refuses the idea of fair competition between social actors who regard each other with suspicion and distrust, act resentfully and selfish, understanding that social opportunities are arbitrary and unpredictable and, when they arise, they should be harnessed by any means, including non-ethical ones.

In a paper from 2012, we argued that the emergence of such a type of individualism is due to the specific mechanisms of communist totalitarianism. We named this type of individualism "survival individualism" (Dascălu 2012, 259), and it appears as a perverse effect of totalitarian collectivism under the influence of specific mechanisms, such as fear or shortage economy. The official communist ideology was a collectivist one in which society, class and group take precedence over the individual. This ideology, however, could not be imposed on all members of socialist society so as to become a genuine belief of all. The new man the communist propaganda spoke of, who shared, among other things, deeply collectivist beliefs, was created only to a small extent. Most subjects of communist power, who were supposed to become perfect subjects, unable to revolt against the regime and ready to fulfil orders from those who held power, in any circumstances, only partly believed in the official ideology. Most people more or less respected the communist ritual without really believing in it. It was more important to "make ends meet," i.e. to achieve one's own interests, regardless of others.

Here's how a collectivist ideology and a socio-economic system based on it produce a perverse effect of individualism. Communism seeks to atomize society and break the traditional ties. Social atoms are easier to control and manipulate than well-established social organizations from the civil society. Continuous surveillance, and the threat of severe repression for non-compliance with the power's requests and the ideological ritual, lead to some duplication of personality, to Orwellian "doublethink" or "double-talk," to the withdrawal of the individual in the small universe of one's family or group of friends, considered to be safer. Continuous threat of shortages of products and services needed to survive, leading to a focus on immediate self-interest in finding the best means to achieve it. Fear and other specific mechanisms of communism break social ties between individuals, whereas the ideological glue that ought to make a whole atomized mass malleable and manipulable is no longer trusted.

To be sure, the perverse effect of communist collectivism, the survival individualism, is likely to overlap the Romanian tradition of individualism that Rădulescu-Motru talked about, enhancing its effects. Obviously, they are in fact new research directions of individualism in former communist countries.

Conclusions

Our research seems to show that students of the Social Work study program are already in possession of a relatively well-defined motivation for choosing the profession, that they have a relatively accurate view of this line of work and their motivation is based on a set of professional values. Altruism, one of these professional values, seems to have become a central one for students, mainly because of what they have learned in school or in practice, and tends to support the future exercise of their profession.

The students' individualism, although situated at a relatively high score, is still slightly ambiguous. There are a number of values the students believe in, which would rather guide towards a collectivist vision of organizations. We believe this is due to a number of factors, some pertaining to tradition, some to the actual situation of students, who, in the majority, have not participated directly in the life of an organization that produces goods or services.

Between altruism and individualism, although both are situated at relatively high rates, there is no association, nor are they contradictory. This, however, is gratifying, given that both altruism and individualism, understood as individualism with humanistic traits rather than social selfishness, form the actual foundation of social work practice. We are therefore of the opinion that, at the level of educational contents, this study program should focus more on the core values underlying social work, including the link between altruism and individualism.

References

Alexiu, T. M. (2011). Valori şi faze ale acţiunii în asistenţa social [Balues and Action Phases in Social Work]. In G. Neamţu (Ed.), T*ratat de asistenţă social*. Iaşi: Polirom.

Chelcea, S. (1994), *Personalitate şi societate în tranziţie* [Personality and Society in Transition]. Bucureşti, Societatea Ştiinţă & Tehnică S.A.

Dascălu, D. I. (2012). Frică politică şi individualism în contextul totalitarismului comunist [Political Fear and Individualism in Communist Totalitarianism]. In A. Stan (Ed.), *Psihologie aplicată: dezvoltare intensivă şi extensivă*. Sibiu: Arhip Art.

Dumond, L. (1983). *Essais sur l'individualisme. Une perspective anthropologique sur l'idéologie moderne* [An Essay on Individualism: An Anthropological View on Modern Ideology]. Paris: Seuil.

Durkheim, É. (1987). *L'individualisme et les intellectuels* [Individualism and Intellectuals]. Paris: Mille et une nuits.

Gavreliuc, A. (2011). *Româniile din România. Individualismul autarhic, tipare valorice transgeneraţionale şi autism social* [Romanias within Romania: Autarchic Individuaism, Transgenerational Value Patterns and Social Autism]. Timişoara: Ed. Universităţii de Vest;

Hofstede, G. (2001), *Culture's Consequences*. London, Sage.

Hofstede, G., Hofstede, G. J. & Minkov, M. (2012). *Culturi şi organizaţii. Softul mental* [Cultures and Organisations: The Mental Soft]. Bucureşti: Humanitas.

Lipovetsky, G. (1983). *L'ère du vide. Essais sur l'individualisme contemporain* [Era of Void: An Essay on Contemporary Individualism]. Paris: Galimard.

Moscovici, S. (Ed.). (1998). *Psihologia socială a relaţiilor cu celălalt* [Social Psychology of the Relationships with the Other]. Iaşi: Polirom.

Rădulescu-Motru, C. (1938). Psihologia poporului român [Psychology of the Romanian People]. *Enciclopedia României I*. Bucureşti: Imprimeria Naţională.

Singly, F. De. (2007). *L'individualisme est un humanisme* [Individualism is Humansm]. Paris: Éditions de l'Aube.

Wosińska, W. (2005). *Psihologia vieţii sociale* [Psychology of Social Life]. Bucureşti: Renaissance.

CHAPTER THREE

VULNERABLE POPULATIONS

For Better or Worse! Work-Family Conflict and Couple's Satisfaction with Life

Delia Vîrgă, Silvia Rusu and Roxana Sârbu

Introduction

In more and more couples, the accumulated stress at work affects the quality of their interpersonal relationships. In recent years, the interest of researchers has focused on the transfer of stress from work to personal life, and the impact of work stress on family satisfaction or, more generally, on life satisfaction. The objective of this chapter is to highlight how stress and tension at work have an impact on people who regularly interact with employees in their personal life, i.e. their partners.

Work-family conflict (WFC) is an actual problem present in both popular journals and scientific publications. Work is part of our lives and contributes to defining our identity. However, work can sometimes be intrusive and interferes with different aspects of our life. Work-family conflict has been defined as a form of inter-role conflict in which the role pressures from work and family domains are mutually incompatible in some respects (Greenhaus & Beutell 1985).

The work family border theory was developed by Clark (2000). The basic idea is that work and family are different areas and aspects, characterized by different values. Sometimes, the transition from one area to another can be achieved in an easy way; sometimes the requirements of the field are different from each other, thus making it more difficult to shift. One of the highlights of this model is that when the domains are similar, flexible boundaries will help the work-family balance, while in situations when the domains are different, strong boundaries appear to be more functional.

Starting from the premise that the boundaries between work and families are weak, many researchers have investigated the relationship between work experiences and the quality of the partner relationship. Thus, previous studies have identified two ways in which demands and labour tensions can affect the family, namely the intra-individual transfer of stress (spill over effect) and inter-individual transfer of stress (crossover effect). The spill over effect refers to reactions experienced in the work domain that are transferred and interfere with the non-work domain for the same individual—intra-individual transfers. On the other hand, the crossover effect is defined as the reaction of individuals to the job stress experienced by those with whom they interact regularly (between individuals). Therefore, within any couple, the demands of the job (stressors) or feelings of burnout (strain) can contribute to the stress and/or strain of their partner (Montgomery et al. 2008).

According to the Job Demands-Resources model (Bakker & Demerouti 2007), job demands consist of those physical, psychological, social and organizational aspects of the job that need to be supported by physical and psychological effort (Bakker, Demerouti & Euwama 2005). A category of job-related factors that generate work-family conflicts refers to stress factors or work requirements that are incompatible with family roles. Among the factors that generate the most stressful work-family conflicts are work overload, pressure of work, reorganization and reduction of activity, or job insecurity.

Workload refers to the tasks that an employee must achieve in order to complete the work in a certain period (Karakütük et al. 2003, in Apaydin 2012). Recently, cross-sectional researches showed that higher demands at work are associated with decreased marital satisfaction. Thus, individual's high workloads or general feeling of work stress are associated with decreased marital satisfaction (Ford, Heinen & Langkamer 2007). Moreover, high levels of workload have been found to predict increased anger in spouses (Schulz et al. 2004).

Job insecurity is defined as the perceived threat of job loss and the worries related to that threat (De Witte 2005). It also implies lack of control and feelings of helplessness, both correlated to a low level of well-being of the individual (De Witte 1999). Research shows a negative relationship between job insecurity and life satisfaction (Lim 1997). In addition, a recent meta-analysis shows that work-related well-being is negatively associated with both job insecurity and life satisfaction (Sverke, Hellgren & Näswall 2002).

Numerous studies have correlated role related stressors, in general, and role conflict, in particular, with a variety of work-related attitudes. Research suggests that work-family conflicts can lead to negative attitudes towards work, such as dissatisfaction with work, increased intentions to leave the organization, or even the actual decision to quit the job (Spector et al. 2007). It is considered that such negative emotions lead to stress which further leads to negative attitudes towards work (Ibid.). Previous studies have shown that high levels of work-family conflict are related to low levels of job satisfaction (Stepanski 2002; Thomas & Ganster 1995; Rice, Frone & McFarlin 1992). Work-family conflict is also associated with the quality of work and marriage, as indicators of well-being (Mauno, Kinnunen & Ruokolainen 2006). In terms of satisfaction with life, Allen et al. (2000) show the existence of significant correlations between work-family conflict and satisfaction with life, marriage or family.

Both job satisfaction and family satisfaction contribute to general life satisfaction (Greenhaus et al. 1997; Judge & Watanabe 1993). Several studies support the idea that satisfaction with life domains accounts for 50% of the variance in life satisfaction, while the effects of different events on life satisfaction are largely mediated by satisfaction with life domains (Andrews & Withey 1976; Hart 1999).

Previous research shows that those couples in which both partners prioritize their work and neglect family obligations at home experience work interference with family life because of the inter-individual stress transmission to the partner (Bakker, Demerouti & Burke 2009). It also shows that for both men and women high job demands trigger a work-family conflict and a lower quality of relationship that can negatively affect the partner's well-being (Shimazu, Bakker & Demerouti 2009). When a wife has to deal with high job demands, this will negatively interfere with their family life and increase their feelings of exhaustion that may be transferred to their partner. When a husband has to deal with high job demands, this will affect their family life and eventually will decrease their level of satisfaction with life, which may be transferred to their partners (Demerouti, Bakker & Schaufeli 2005).

This study had two exploratory objectives:

- to examine the effect of spill over on couples, specifically the correlations between job demands and life satisfaction in male and female partners
- to identify the associations between the job demands perceived by one partner and the life satisfaction reported by the other (crossover effect).

Methods

Participants

The participants in this study were 60 dual-earner couples (120 participants) recruited voluntarily under the auspices of an academic research project. The men were slightly older than the women (M_{Men}=37.23 years, M_{Women}=34.68 years). The length of the relationship varied between 15 and 444 months, with a mean duration of 146 months (approximately 12 years). As for the number of children, 60% had at least one child, while 40% did not have any children.

Measures

Work-family conflict was measured with the Negative Work Home Interference Nijmegen scale from the SWING questionnaire (Geurt et al. 2005). The scale contains eight items related to the work-family conflict relationship. The participants were asked to indicate the extent to which their own work negatively influenced the home situation: "How often do you not fully enjoy the company of your spouse/family/friends because you worry about your work?" and "How often do you find it difficult to fulfil your domestic obligations because you are constantly thinking about your work?" (1=never, 5=always). Participants were also requested to indicate the extent to which their partners' work negatively influenced family life. The items were adapted such that they referred to the partner (Bakker, Demerouti & Dollard 2008): "How often does your partner not fully enjoy the company of your spouse/family/friends because you worry about your work," and "How often does your partner find it difficult to fulfil their domestic obligations because they are constantly thinking about work?" (1=never, 5=always). On our sample, Cronbach's alpha was .83 for self-report and .76 for partner's work-family conflict evaluations.

Job insecurity was measured with the four-items version (Staufenbiel & König 2010) of Borg's cognitive job insecurity scale that focuses exclusively on the perception of the likelihood of losing one's job. Some sample items are "My job is secure," "In my opinion I will keep my job in the near future." For the scale we used a Likert response scale ranging from 1 to 5, where (1) means strongly disagree, and (5) means strongly agree. On our sample, Cronbach's alpha was .91.

Workload was measured with five items from the Questionnaire on the Experience and Evaluation of Work (van Veldhoven et al. 2002). Items were answered on a five point Likert-type scale ranging from 1=never to

5=always. A sample item is: "Do you experience a heavy workload?" (on our sample, Cronbach's alpha=.82)

Satisfaction with life was measured using the five-item Satisfaction with Life Scale (Diener et al. 1985). Some sample items are "In most ways my life is close to my ideal," "The conditions of my life are excellent," "I am satisfied with my life." Items were rated on a seven-point Likert scale (1=strongly disagree, 7=strongly agree). On our sample, Cronbach's alpha was .86.

Satisfaction with relationship with partner was also measured by a single item: "How satisfied are you with your partner relationship?" The participants answered this question on a Likert scale ranging from 1 to 5, (1=very dissatisfied, 5=very satisfied).

Job satisfaction was measured by a single item: "How satisfied are you with your job?" The participants answered this question on a Likert scale ranging from 1 to 5, (1=very dissatisfied, 5=very satisfied).

Procedure

The participants were informed that all the data provided would be confidential and used for research purposes only, after which participants answered the paper-pencil version of the questionnaires.

Results

Spill over effect among female employees

For the first objective Table 3-1 and 3-2 demonstrate the statistical results. In Table 3-1, we present the correlations between job demands and different types of satisfaction reported by female employees as partners.

Table 3-1. Correlations between variables measured among women

Variables	1	2	3	4	5	6	7
1. F_WFC perceived in partner	--						
2. F_WFC self-reported	**.48***	--					
3. F_Job Insecurity	-.21	-.13	--				
4. F_Workload	.07	**.43***	**-.26***	--			
5. F_life satisfaction	-.17	-.10	.06	.10	--		
6. F_relationship satisfaction	**-.35***	-.12	-.13	.11	**.50***	--	
7. F_job satisfaction	-.19	**-.42***	.10	**-.31***	.18	.12	--

N=60, * for p < .05

As we can see in Table 3-1 above, the workload perceived is positively associated with the WFC reported by the women (r=.43, p < .01). Women who perceive a high level of their own WFC also report a lower job satisfaction (r=- .42, p < .01), while women's perception of their partner's WFC is negatively associated with relationship satisfaction (r=-.35, p < .01). These results support the idea of a spill over effect on women employees for two types of job demands: workload and work-family conflict. Moreover, another argument to support the spill over effect is the positive correlation between life satisfaction and relationship satisfaction among women (r=.50, p < .01).

Spill over effect among male employees

In Table 3-2 below we present the correlations between job demands and different types of satisfaction reported by male employees as partners.

As we can see, men who perceive a high level of job insecurity also report a lower level of relationship satisfaction (r=-.30, p < .01). The workload reported by men is positively associated with the self-reported level of WFC (r=.40, p < .01). Men who consider their partner as having a high WFC report a lower level of life satisfaction (r=-.30, p < .01). These results support the idea of a spill over effect among male employees for two types of job demands: job insecurity and workload. For men, the perception of their partner's level of work-family conflict is important for their life satisfaction. Furthermore, another argument for the spill over effect is the positive correlation between life satisfaction and relationship satisfaction among men, and between job satisfaction and life satisfaction.

Table 3-2. Correlations between variables measured among men

Variables	1	2	3	4	5	6	7
1. M_WFC perceived in partner	--						
2. M_WFC self-reported	**48***	--					
3. M_Job insecurity	-.02	.12	--				
4. M_Workload	02	**.40***	.22	--			
5. M_life satisfaction	**-.30***	.01	-.10	.01	--		
6. M_relationship satisfaction	-.04	-.03	**-.30***	-.15	**.28***	--	
7. M_job satisfaction	-.19	-.08	.14	-.05	**.39***	.17	--

N=60, * for $p < .05$

Crossover effect from female to male employees

For the second objective, the correlation matrices of the research variables can be found in Tables 3-3 and 3-4 below. In Table 3-3, we present the correlations between job demands perceived by women and different types of satisfaction reported by men as partners.

As we can see in Table 3-3, the self-reported WFC of women is negatively associated with their partner's level of job satisfaction ($r=-.31$, $p < .01$), and life satisfaction ($r=-.25$, $p < .05$). Thus, the crossover effect was present from women to men, in the investigated couples, as shown by the work-family conflict perceived by women and its impact on the job and life satisfaction of men.

Table 3-3. Correlations between variables among men and women

Variables	1	2	3	4	5	6	7
1. F_WFC perceived in partner	--						
2. F_WFC self-report	**.48***	--					
3. F_Job insecurity	-.21	-.13	--				
4. F_Workload	.07	**.43***	**-.26***	--			
5. M_life satisfaction	-.20	**-.25***	.00	.04	--		.
6. M_relationship satisfaction	-.23	-.02	-.05	.07	**.28***	--	
7. M_job satisfaction	**-.25***	**-.31***	.10	-.14	**.39***	.17	

N=60, * for p < .05

Crossover effect from men to women employees

In Table 3-4, we present the correlations between job demands perceived by men and different types of satisfaction reported by women as couples.

Table 3-4. Correlations between variables among men and women

Variables	1	2	3	4	5	6	7
1. M_WFC perceived in partner	--						
2. M_WFC self-reported	**.48***	--					
3. M_Job_insecurity	-.02	.12	--				
4. M_Workload	.02	**.40***	.22	--			
5. F_life satisfaction	-.09	.12	-.11	.15	--		
6. F_relationship satisfaction	-.05	-.03	**-.27***	-.01	**.50***	--	
7. F_job satisfaction	-.13	.17	.04	**.25***	.18	.12	--

N=60, * for p < .05

As we can see in Table 3-4, the level of workload reported by men is positively associated with their partner's job satisfaction (r=.25, $p < .05$). Moreover, when men perceive a high level of job insecurity, their spouses are less satisfied with the relationship with their partner (r=-.27, $p< .05$). Thus, the crossover effect was present from men to women in investigated couples, specifically regarding the job insecurity perceived by men and its impact on the satisfaction felt by women concerning their partner relationship.

Conclusion

On a general level, our findings suggest that spill over and crossover effects are present in dual-earner couples. Thus, the work-family conflict perceived by the women is negatively associated with job and partner satisfaction. Job insecurity perceived by men is negatively associated with their relationship satisfaction. Work-family conflict perceived by the women is negatively associated with job and life satisfaction in men. Job insecurity perceived by men can make them neglect the relationship with their partner, which can explain a lower level of relationship satisfaction reported by the female partners.

Our study has some limitations. We collected data from a relatively small convenience sample. A larger number of couples and a longitudinal design of a future study can offer the possibility to investigate causal effects. Another future direction to develop the study could be to explore moderator variables in the relationship between job demands and life satisfaction (e.g. job satisfaction could be one of these moderators). Furthermore, the crossover and spill over of positive experiences should receive more research attention. There are already some studies showing how positive experiences like work engagement can have a positive impact on partner's wellbeing (Bakker, Demerouti & Schaufeli 2005), but further research should investigate the mechanisms supporting this positive crossover, and how it can be enhanced.

This information can be used successfully by managers and human resources specialists in the development of management strategies that lead to the creation, development and implementation of a healthy work environment in organizations. The balance between work and personal life can be achieved by finding and maintaining a balance between the rhythm of the career and personal responsibilities.

References

Allen, T. D., Herst, D. E., Bruck, C. S. & Sutton, M. (2000). Consequences associated with work-to family conflict: a review and agenda for future research. *Journal of Occupational Health Psychology 5*: 278-308.

Andrews, F. A. & Withey, S. B (1976). *Social indicators of well-being in America: The development and measurement of perceptual indicators*. New York, NY: Plenum Press.

Apaydin, C. (2012). The Workload of Faculty Members: The Example of Educational Faculties in Turkey. *College Student Journal 46*: 203-213.

Bakker, A. B. & Demerouti, E. (2007). The Job Demands-Resources model: State of the art. *Journal of Managerial Psychology 22*: 309-328.

Bakker, A. B., Demerouti, E. & Burke, R. (2009). Workaholism and relationship quality: A spill over-crossover perspective. *Journal of Occupational Health Psychology 14*: 23-33.

Bakker, A. B., Demerouti, E. & Dollard, F. M. (2008). How Job Demands Affect Partners' Experience of Exhaustion: Integrating Work–Family Conflict and Crossover Theory. *Journal of Applied Psychology 93*: 901-911.

Bakker, A. B., Demerouti, E. & Euwema, M. (2005). Job Resources Buffer the Impact of Job Demands on Burnout. *Journal of Occupational Health Psychology 10*: 170-180.

Bakker, A. B., Demerouti, E. & Schaufeli, W. B. (2005). The crossover of burnout and work engagement among working couples. *Human Relations 58 (5)*: 661-689.

Clark, S. C. (2000). Work-family border theory: A new theory of work-family balance. *Human Relations 53 (6)*: 747-770.

De Witte, H. (1999). Job insecurity and psychological well-being: Review of the literature and exploration of some unresolved issues. *European Journal of Work and Organizational Psychology*, *8*(2), 155-177.

—. (2005). Job insecurity: Review of the international literature on definitions, prevalence, antecedents and consequences. *SA Journal of Industrial Psychology 31*: 1-6.

Demerouti, E., Bakker, B. A. & Schaufeli B. W. (2005). Spill over and crossover of exhaustion and life satisfaction among dual-earner parents. *Journal of Vocational Behavior 67*: 266-289.

Diener, E., Oishi, S. & Lucas, E.R. (2003). Personality, culture, and subjective well-being: Emotional and Cognitive Evaluations of Life. *Annu. Rev. Psychol. 54*: 403-25

Ford, M. T., Heinen, B. A. & Langkamer, K. L. (2007). Work and family satisfaction and conflict: A meta-Analysis of cross-domain relations. *Journal of Applied Psychology 92*: 57-80.

Greenhaus, J. H. & Beutell, N. J. (1985). Sources of conflict between work and family roles. *The Academy of Management Review 10*: 76-88.

Greenhaus, J. H., Collins, K. M., Singh, R. & Parasuraman, S. (1997). Work and family influences on departure from public accounting. *Journal of Vocational Behavior 50 (2)*: 249-270.

Hart, P. M. (1999). Predicting employee life satisfaction: A coherent model of personality, work, and nonwork experiences, and domain satisfactions. *Journal of Applied Psychology 84 (4)*: 564.

Judge, T. A. & Watanabe, S. (1993). Another look at the job–life satisfaction relationship. *Journal of Applied Psychology*, *78*, 939-948.

Lim, V. (1997). Moderating effects of work-based support on the relationship between job insecurity and its consequences. *Work & Stress 11 (3)*: 251-266.

Mauno, S., Kinnunen, U. & Ruokolainen, M. (2006). Exploring work- and organization-based resources as moderators between work-family conflict, well-being, and job attitudes. *Work & Stress 20 (3)*: 210-233.

Montgomery, J. A., Peeters, C. W. M., Schaufeli, B. W. & Panagopoulou, P., E. (2008). Crossover and work-home interference. *The Irish Journal of Psychology 29*: 61-76.

Rice, R. W., Frone, M. R. & McFarlin, D. B. (1992). Work-nonwork conflict and the perceived quality of life. *Journal of Organizational Behaviour* 13: 155-168.

Schulz, M. S., Cowan, P. A., Cowan, C. P. & Brennan, R. T. (2004). Coming home upset: Gender, marital satisfaction, and the daily spill over of work experience into couple interaction. *Journal of Family Psychology 18*: 250-263.

Shimazu, A., Bakker, B. A. & Demerouti, E. (2009). How job demands affect an intimate partner: a test of the spill over-crossover model in Japan. *Journal of Occupational Health 51*: 239-248.

Spector, P. E., Allen, T. D., Poelmans, S. A. Y., LaPierre, L. M., Cooper, C. L., O'Driscoll, M., Sanchez, J. I., Abarca, N., Alexandrova, M., Beham, B., Brough, P., Ferreiro, P., Fraile, G., Lu, C. Q., Lu, L., Moreno-Velasquez, I., Pagon, M., Pitariu, H., Salamatov, V., Shima, S., Siminoni, A. S., Siu, O. L. & Widerszal-Bazyl, M. (2007). Cross-national differences in relationships of work demands, job satisfaction, and turnover intentions with work-family conflict. *Personnel Psychology 60 (4)*: 805-835.

Staufenbiel, T. & König, C. J. (2010). A model for the effects of job insecurity on performance, turnover intention, and absenteeism. *Journal of Occupational and Organizational Psychology 83 (1)*: 101-117.

Stepanski, K. M. (2002). *Work-family conflict theories: Integration and model development*. Unpublished dissertation. Wayne State University.

Sverke, M., Hellgren, J. & Näswall, K. (2002). No security: A meta-analysis and review of job insecurity and its consequences. *Journal of Occupational Health Psychology 7(3)*: 242-264.

Thomas, L. T. & Ganster, D. C. (1995). Impact of family-supportive work variables on on work-family conflict and strain: A control perspective. *Journal of Applied Psychology 80*: 6-15.

Van Veldhoven, M., De Jong, J., Broersen, S., Kompier, M. & Meijman, Y. (2002). Specific relationships between psychosocial job conditions and job related stress: a three-level analytic approach. *Work and Stress 16*, 207-228.

Westman, M. (2006). Crossover of stress and strain in the work-family context. In Mina Westman, Fiona Jones & Ronald J. Burke (Eds.), *Work-life balance: A psychological perspective*. New York, NY: Psychology Press. 163-184.

OVERCOMING PROBLEM BEHAVIOUR AND HELPING AUTISTIC CHILDREN TO COMMUNICATE

LAURA-CRISTINA OPRICA

Introduction

The topic for this chapter hasn't been chosen at random; in fact, there are many discussions on this theme and it has become intensely debated as teachers are receiving more and more pupils with autism in their language classes. As autism includes problematic behaviour, the topic seems even more important. On a daily basis, every teacher has at his or her disposal a range of solutions when students behave disruptively or uncooperatively.

For me and most teachers, an effective way to get past such unpleasant situations is to use clearly agreed sanctions, keeping in mind to focus and criticize the behaviour and not the student. Still, in many situations these strategies fall short of the mark, despite all our best efforts, and we have to talk in private about what has happened with those students who are reluctant to follow the established rules (Harmer 2007).

However, when teachers have to work with autistic children they feel that problem behaviour needs to be somehow re-defined and creating a successful learning environment requires more patience, self control and imagination than any other teaching situation.

This chapter aims to bring attention to some methods and techniques designed especially to help teachers and parents who find themselves crossing such unfamiliar territory. Apart from this, throughout the pages you are about to read I am going to highlight some of the problems autistic children have to overcome in my country and what kind of support the educational system offers.

Nevertheless, I cannot move forward to discuss the matters stated above without taking a brief moment to consider why autism is still unknown to the vast majority of people. Perhaps it is due to the fact that nobody has managed to explain exactly why this disability occurs and find once and for all a complete definition. It seems that years and years of research have gathered pieces of information about what autism is not, rather than making it clear what it is.

Briefly said, autism is a lifelong developmental disability that affects the way a person relates to other people and hinders communication. A child or an adult avoiding contact and interaction and living in a world of their own is usually the most commonly understood portrait people have, demonstrated whenever they are asked to describe in a sentence what autism is all about. I find it important to highlight that autism is a spectrum condition, meaning that certain difficulties will be shared by everyone who has been diagnosed with this disability.

However, these difficulties may appear and affect certain individuals in different ways (Whitaker 2001). So far, in my teaching career I have met several children with the same deficiency. Nevertheless, they have their own profile of abilities, skills and, of course, their own personalities which we should take into account. Experience and learning help to develop their character and I have noticed a huge difference in accepting behaviour norms when teachers find the right solutions to work with these children.

Unfortunately, as it is a neurological disorder and is not triggered by any environmental factors or induced in some other way, we have no possibility of putting an end to it (Teisten 2010). Our best option is treatment, and although many case studies have helped to ease the lives of those affected, no cure has been found. Leaving aside such details which might prove more helpful for doctors, the next section sheds more light on the educational challenge every teacher has to face when working with autistic children.

Methods and Techniques

Teachers find it difficult and challenging to teach children with autism because everything we know about learning and student behaviour is turned upside down and becomes inconsistent. I think we all agree that children tend to follow a similar path as far as their intellectual development is concerned. Certainly, some children tend to work faster than others, but all in all these various rates are within normal range.

Children with autism have their own peculiar styles of communication and developing interpersonal relationships that seem to follow an unknown path (Quill 1995). To be able to develop strategies meant to work and promote communication and social integration we have to understand these differences and incorporate them into intervention. It is true that the earlier a child receives specialized help the more likely he or she is to overcome disabilities.

We have to bear in mind that we can encounter students with severe learning difficulties who make very little social contact, but also children of average intelligence who are fluent but may simply exhibit some unconventional mannerisms. Speaking of problem behaviour, it is true that it is more difficult to work with such children, but difficult does not mean impossible, and it certainly does not have to mean useless.

What most teachers have found particularly hard to understand is why a certain student would behave in a particular way. Without knowing what lies behind an aggressive or odd behaviour nobody can control the situation. Perhaps teachers should be talking about methods and techniques used, but how can anyone aim to teach something without the right conditions to do so?

As I have seldom noticed, the problem is such children are not able to express their feelings due to their limited verbal communication. So, frustration, anxiety, fear, stress or discomfort might pile up slowly until they eventually reach the surface in an outburst of unwanted behaviour.

Therefore, no matter which method we are thinking of applying, it is important to reduce their level of stress and anxiety before any sign of communication can be seen. I said communication rather than learning because at the lowest levels better communication is always the aim.

The problem is that these children already have some major language issues and it seems that their mother tongue is a foreign one. So how can we teach them English? A world-renowned autism expert, Ivar Lovaas, gave everyone an answer when he said: “If they can’t learn the way we teach, we teach the way they learn.”

To begin with, we should use short instructions in the foreign language and whenever it is possible we should come up with some kind of visual support (Myers & Burnett 2004). In fact, the usage of complex instructions is never useful, because even our best students might get bored before we even start the exercise.

Teaching English also proves to be a difficult task, because most students have a literal understanding of words and phrases and despite all our efforts they cannot see past that particular meaning. The answer to a simple phrase such as “Can you show me your identity card?” took me aback. The answer was “I cannot. My identity card is in my wallet.” A good way to solve this and make them understand what you mean is to switch roles—while the student asks for the identity card, the teacher presents it. Then, for better comprehension, the roles may be switched as many times as we think is necessary.

On the positive side, these children like routine, role playing and lots of repetition. Speaking of repetition, even healthy grown ups occasionally repeat what others say without fully understanding the meaning because it is a good strategy to learn a language. Kids with autism tend to use this technique almost exclusively and we can take advantage of this. Learning grammar, set phrases, numbers and vocabulary will turn into a fun activity as long as we keep in mind to bring forward what is best in our students and what fits their learning style. Trying to find differences between them and other students is a pointless task and work in vain.

Teaching students how to combine the words they keep repeating in original sentences is one more challenge to overcome and probably the hardest. For some particular students I worked with memory was their strong point, so to begin with we learnt little scripts combining more and more grammar every day.

I always thought it is not enough to teach children what a word means. As I always tell my students: “You cannot go to a shop with a vocabulary list. Make sure you are able to make up some simple sentences in order to let people know what you need.” We have to do our best to teach them to have useful conversations, to comment upon the things they see around them and to express their feelings (Saltzman & Kelly 2010). Whether we face it or not, everybody longs to be accepted and acceptance for an autistic person will be gained when they are able to communicate and step closer to our world.

It is also the teacher’s responsibility to design activities that teach both receptive and expressive language. What a child understands is called receptive language, but what a child says, on the other hand, is called expressive language. Before any activity is thought of, teachers should devote energy and time to form a relationship.

It is wrong to say that we have to talk in order to communicate and bond. The tone of your voice, the way you look and your body language might help you get closer to a student, or on the contrary push you further away (Myers & Burnett 2004).

By far the most difficult task teachers have is to work with a child who does not make visual contact. Without students looking at us, it is more difficult to pick up their nonverbal cues, and sooner or later they are going to feel upset and ignored. Therefore, in one situation I had to analyze what was going on before the outburst to make a connection. Later on, I was told by the parents that such behaviour usually reached its purpose and the child got what they wanted.

As a general rule, and from personal experience, it is important to be consistent in the way you interact with such a student and also consistent when you have to deal with challenging behaviour. Not every child suffering from autism has a problematic behaviour, and even if this kind of behaviour appears it does not mean that it will become a feature throughout their life.

When communication is no longer an issue, teachers should encourage response, use clear and precise language, clearly structured tasks and encourage interaction with others, although we should first be open to accepting solitary work.

Visual aids and roleplay activities have so far worked well with students I have worked with, at least as a starting point. I also brought in pictures to teach the names of different objects. By constantly repeating what that object was, some children were gradually able to exchange a picture for the desired object.

Discussions

Up until now, we as teachers have had plenty of opportunities to work with autistic children, but to be honest we wanted the conditions to be somewhat different. Unfortunately, my country has not developed enough programs to help these children, and those which are running are not widely available. Every method explained above has been used in regular schools by many teachers.

Unfortunately, just as many autistic children are sent to normal schools, although they clearly need specialized help. But where to get this help? The city in which I live has only one school for these children. The school for which I work has few qualified teachers to help its children in need (by qualified I mean that there are teachers who know what autism is and have adjusted their expectations accordingly).

Sadly, for the rural area we have to work in, compromises have to be made. Although nobody likes this situation, the children there have only two options: come and join a public, regular school or stay at home with no education at all. A lack of solutions and financial support combined with indifference is more than enough to let things go on, as if nothing is wrong.

Of course, as teachers we cannot pretend those children do not exist. We do our best to provide different tasks, but with at least twenty children in a class, how much time can we dedicate to one or two autistic children? Most teachers would answer "not enough," and anyone who has been in this kind of situation understands why we are saying this.

Therapy cannot be complete in a regular school and English teaching is even more difficult because it requires many visual aids, special materials and a lot of communicative activities. Before discussing a few ideas about communicative activities there are some things which should be said about teaching materials. Unfortunately, the schools located in the rural areas have only one textbook between every two children, so you can imagine that learning a foreign language is hard in these conditions.

Usually, the other children in the class do not understand why their colleague gets different tasks. They also wonder why some teachers spend more time talking with children who do not answer back or cannot repeat a simple word.

Children are known to be cruel, especially when they are young, so the relationship between an autistic child and the rest of the class is bound to be tense. Do you still wonder what this has to do with English teaching? Well, especially at low levels, we use a lot of pair and group work to liven up the atmosphere and learn cooperation and communication. In most cases, children refuse to work with a child who they have already tagged as being different from them, and therefore bonds cannot be established.

From what I have observed, the relationship between the autistic child and the others is a tense one. First, it is a problematic relationship because autism implies unusual social communication. These children do not know how to behave around other children, so most of the time they appear rude or selfish.

Talking with parents I have tried to explain early intervention matters, because the brain is vulnerable in early life and can mould itself to the environment it initially faces. However, some of them lack the financial support they need, while some have embraced acceptance. They are not used to the idea of celebrating small successes and they keep comparing their child to other children. This happens especially if, at home, they have two or three children who behave in a normal way.

I even heard parents saying that they like having a special child and they do not wish to change them. What they do not realize is that the important thing here is not trying to change someone. Due to the fact that those kids are indeed special, we have to change our way of doing things and the first phrase to get rid of is "this child will never be able to do that."

Of course, autism implies some limitations, but this does not mean we have to jump to conclusions before trying to do something about the matter. Nobody wishes to say that those parents do not love their children; the problem is that they are far too judgemental and chances are that the other children they are raising will take after them.

Conclusions

Many things have been said up until now about autism, but it seems like the general attention has shifted and people are trying to find methods to cope with this disability instead of trying to find a cure. It is indeed a good strategy, at least for the moment, to improve what we cannot change.

However, in the country in which I live, too much time and money has been wasted in designing projects to help the autistic, and sadly these projects have been cancelled or forgotten along the way. Some schools were opened but only in large cities, and as I have witnessed myself there is greater demand than available places.

Besides this, there are not enough training courses available. There should be courses to create specialized teachers and courses to help parents. Especially in the rural areas, parents learn from the teachers working in schools to help their child. In turn, most of us have learnt strategies to work with these children from the internet or from books. Teachers' lack of knowledge about autism is another sad topic. Turning in incomplete assignments, disobeying the teacher and not answering questions might be more than enough reason to form a long-lasting negative opinion about a student who in fact needs help, rather than someone to criticize his or her every step.

So what should be done? Obviously, we need to be aware of the fact that we do not have enough programs and should do something to change this. When things are set on the right track efforts should be made to educate and inform the general public about this disability. What chances does an autistic child in Romania have to learn a foreign language? What chances does an autistic child have in general? The answer to these questions is little chance, close to none. Ironically enough, it is a matter of luck for these children. Everybody deserves the right to have an education and it seems that in our modern society those who have the power to change something have forgotten this.

References

Feisten, A. (2010). *A History of Autism: Conversation with the Pioneeers.* Hoboken, NJ: Wiley-Blackwell.

Harmer, J. (2007). *The Practice of English Language Teaching.* Harlow: Pearson Longman.

Myers, J. & Burnett, C. (2004). *Teaching English. The Essential Guide for Teachers.* London: Bloomsbury Academic.

Quill, K. A. (1995). *Teaching Children with Autism. Strategies to Enhance Communication and Socialization.* Stamford, CT: Cengage Learning.

Saltzman, M. & Kelly, K. (2010). *A Behavioral Approach to Teaching Language. What It Is and Why It's Useful.* 26-32.

Whitaker, P. (2001). *Challenging Behaviour and Autism: Making Sense—Making Progress*. Shawnee Mission, KS: Autism Asperger Publishing Company.

PREVALENCE OF INTESTINAL GIARDIASIS IN INSTITUTIONALIZED ELDERLY PATIENTS

IOSIF MARINCU, IOANA TODOR AND MIHAI MAREŞ

Introduction

Giardiasis is a widespread parasitic condition, caused by the flagellated protozoa *Giardia lamblia*, also known as *Giardia intestinalis* or *Giardia duodenalis.* This disease is considered the most common cosmopolitan bowel parasitosis, encountered in highly developed countries, as well as developing and underdeveloped countries (Hawrelak 2003, 129).

International studies estimate a figure of 2.8×10^6 human infections per year with this ubiquitous parasite that causes diarrhoea and nutritional deficits, most frequently in children, but also in adults from all over the world (Syed 2003, 453).

Many specialists have proven that the prevalence of giardiasis is directly associated with the socio-economic status of the population as well as with the health education and climate conditions in respective areas. Thus, in North American countries with a very high economic level, the medium prevalence of giardiasis is merely 1.4% of the general population. On the other hand, in underdeveloped South American countries the prevalence of giardiasis is 24%, and this region is considered a high risk area for this common parasitosis (Julio 2012, 11).

This small bowel parasite can create endemic areas or isolated cases of food or water poisoning, manifesting nausea, vomiting, diarrhoea, malabsorption syndrome, dehydration syndrome, loss of weight, lipid malabsorption, vitamin B12 deficit, anaemia, and even chronic diarrhoea (Hawrelak 2003, 129; Syed 2003, 453).

The prevalence of intestinal parasites is a direct consequence of a set of constant factors, particularly climate, food and water supplies, personal and community hygiene, sanitation, proximity to both domestic and wild animals, and socioeconomic conditions that play an important role in the stages of the epidemiologic and physiopatologic processes of this widespread parasitosis (Julio 2012, 12).

The high incidence worldwide, ranging between 20 and 60% (Hawrelak 2003, 129), as well as the general unbalance with serious nutritional and multiple vitamin deficiencies, has generated several studies concerning the physiopathologic mechanisms of this condition, its risk factors and means of treatment to reduce specific morbidity in children and adults alike (Syed 2003, 453). The aim of our study is to estimate the prevalence of intestinal lambliasis in elderly patients admitted in various institutions throughout Timiş County.

Methods

We retrospectively analyzed a group of 48 elderly patients that were admitted to the Infectious Diseases Clinic in Timisoara for various conditions. They all came from nursing homes in Timisoara, Buzias, Peciu Nou, Varias and from the Psychiatric Hospitals in Gataia and Jebel.

The positive diagnosis was determined based on subjective clinical features (anorexia, fatigue, abdominal discomfort, cramps, flatulence, nausea, stomach pain, liver pain, headaches, etc.) and objective features (hepatomegalia, non-specific skin eruptions, eczematous dermatitis, loss of weight, etc.), correlated with biological tests (white cell count, coproparasitologic examination, natremia, kalemia, calcemia, etc.).

In all patients, coproparasitologic exams were performed every 1–2 days in order to diagnose digestive lambliasis. This examination (the Lugol method) consists of two steps of the macroscopic and microscopic evaluation of faeces obtained from our study subjects. All the procedures were performed in the Bacteriology Laboratory of the Dr. Victor Babes Infectious Diseases and Pneumophtisiology Hospital in Timisoara. Statistical data was processed with the Epi Info software.

Results

Twenty-eight (58.33%) patients were men and 20 (41.66%) women, with an average age of 71 (ranging from 60 to 85). Because of low immunity and life in institutionalized communities, the elderly are exposed to a number of infections of bacterial, viral and parasitic aetiology. We admitted and clinically monitored 26 (54.16%) patients with acute enterocolitis, 12 (25%) patients with acute pneumonia, 6 (12.5%) patients with chronic hepatitis, 2 (4.1%) patients with liver cirrhosis, and 2 (4.1%) patients with acute bronchopneumonia.

Their individual data and medical history are well-known factors that can change the evolution and prognosis of acute infections in the elderly. In our group we found numerous coexisting conditions: 26 patients treated for chronic ischemic cardiopathy, 20 patients treated for hypertension, 18 patients with cardiac failure, 9 patients with diabetes, 19 patients with obesity, 11 patients with chronic duodenal ulcer, 18 patients with gall-bladder litiasis, 4 patients with asthma, 6 patients with liver cirrhosis, 13 patients with chronic alcoholism, 4 patients with psoriasis, 8 patients with various neoplasms, and 4 patients with chronic kidney failure (see Table 3-5 below).

Table 3-5. Coexisting conditions

Comorbidities	Patients	
	No	%
Chronic ischemic cardiopathy	26	54.16%
Hypertension	20	41.66%
Heart failure	18	37.50%
Diabetes	9	18.75%
Obesity	19	39.58%
Duodenal ulcer	11	22.91%
Gull-bladder litiasis	18	37.50%
Asthma	4	8.33%
OCBP	6	12.50%
Viral chronic hepatitis	5	10.41%
Liver cirrhosis	6	12.50%
Chronic kidney failure	4	8.33%
Chronic alcoholism	13	27.08%
Neoplasms	8	16.66%
Psoriasis	4	8.33%

Following biological and paraclinical examinations, 34 (70.83%) of the 48 patients were found harbouring *Giardia lamblia* cysts. Aside from the symptoms for which they were admitted, all of the patients showed clinical and objective changes that could guide the physician towards a diagnostic of giardiasis: prolonged diarrhoea (76.47%), stomach cramps (70.58%), postprandial bloating (94.11%), flatulence (97.05%), nausea (88.23%), vomiting (44.11%), pyrosis (88.23%), bitter taste in the morning (94.11%), burping (88.23%), foul breath (82.35%), stomach pain (88.23%), lack of appetite (94.11%). Some of the non-digestive complaints, such as neuropsychic or allergic, are: headache (97.05%), marked asthenia (100%), paresthesia in the lower limbs (73.52%), restlessness (35.29%), irritability (52.94%), insomnia (76.47%), drowsiness (41.17%), depression (82.35%), and prurigo (44.11%). The objective examination revealed the following changes: skin pallor (94.11%), eczematous dermatitis (35.29%), persistent skin fold (70.58%), dry skin (76.47%), skin rashes (41.17%), bowel distension (88.23%), and loss of weight (35.29%) (see Table 3-6 below).

Table 3-6. Reported symptoms and physical signs

Symptoms	Cases No	%	Clinical signs	Cases No	%
Diarrhoea	26	76.47%	Skin pallor	32	94.11%
Abdominal cramps	24	70.58%	Eczematous dermatitis	12	35.29%
Postprandial bloating	32	94.11%	Persistent skin fold	24	70.58%
Flatulence	33	97.05%	Dry skin	26	76.47%
Nausea	30	88.23%	Skin rashes	14	41.17%
Vomiting	15	44.11%	Abdominal distension	30	88.23%
Cirrhosis	30	88.23%	Weight loss	12	35.29%
Bitter taste in the morning	32	94.11%			
Burping	30	88.23%			
Bad breath	28	82.35%			
Epigastric pain	30	88.23%			
Headache	33	97.05%			
Loss of appetite	32	94.11%			
Asthenia	34	100.00%			
Paresthesia	25	73.52%			
Restlessness	12	35.29%			
Irritability	18	52.94%			
Insomnia	26	76.47%			
Drowsiness	14	41.17%			
Depression	28	82.35%			
Prurigo	15	44.11%			

Finding the cause of diarrhoea is an important step in starting the right therapy. In our group, we were able to identify the causing agent in only 21 of the 26 patients, while 5 remained undetermined. Using the coproparasitologic examination, we identified 17 patients with *Giardia lamblia,* 2 patients with *Salmonella*, 1 patient with *Staphylococcus aureus*, and 1 patient with *Escherichia coli* (see Table 3-7 below).

Table 3-7. Etiologic agents in patients with diarrhoea

Etiologic agent	Patients	
	No	%
Staphylococcus aureus	1	3.84%
Salmonella	2	7.69%
Escherichia coli	1	3.84%
Giardia lamblia	17	65.38%

In massive infections with *Giardia* there are important absorption deficiencies for the main food constituents (proteins, lipids, carbohydrates) some vitamins (vitamin A, vitamin B complex), and iron, calcium, magnesium, etc. Some of the biological changes in patients with giardiasis are anaemia (26 patients), eosinophilia (28 patients), hypogammaglobulinemia (14 patients), hypoproteinemia (12 patients), hyponatremia (15 patients), hypocalcaemia (18 patients), hypomagnesaemia (16 patients), and hypokalemia (12 patients) (see Table 3-8 below).

Table 3-8. Biological changes in patients with giardiasis

Biological changes	Patients	
	No	%
Anaemia	26	76.47%
Eosinophilia	28	82.35%
Hypogammaglobulinemia	14	41.17%
Hypoproteinemia	12	35.29%
Hyponatremia	15	44.11%
Hypocalcaemia	18	52.94%
Hypomagnesaemia	16	47.05%
Hypokalemia	12	35.29%

Clinically manifested giardiasis may evolve as an acute condition, with acute diarrhoea, or as a chronic condition, with chronic diarrhoea, malabsorption syndrome and weight loss. Seventeen (50%) of the 34 patients with giardiasis had acute diarrhoea, 3 (8.82%) had chronic diarrhoea, and 6 (17.64%) had alternating diarrhoea and constipation (see Figure 3-1 below).

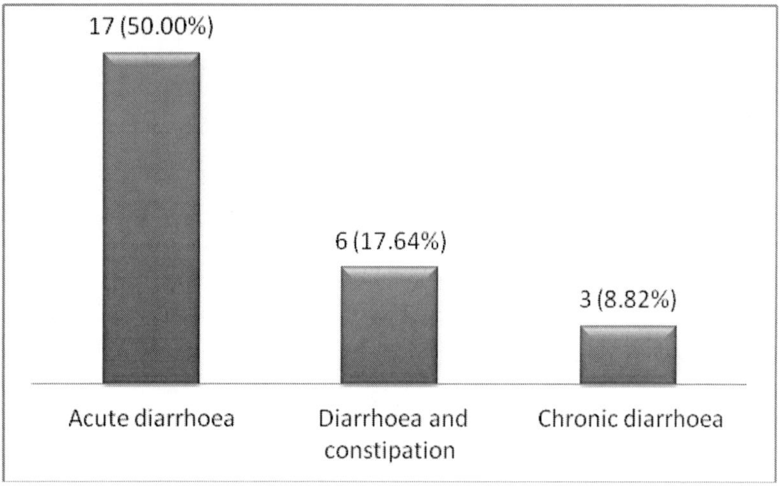

Figure 3-1. Clinical aspects of giardiasis

All patients diagnosed with giardiasis were administered two tablets of Albendazole (Zentel, 200 mg) per day, for five days, along with symptomatic medication (analgesics, antispastics, calcium, omeprazole, vitamin B complex, etc.). The clinical evolution was favourable, with no unusual adverse reactions. Coproparasitologic examination was negative at the end of treatment in all 30 tested patients. We have to underline that 26 of the 34 patients needed hydro-electrolytic restoration using Ringer solution, glucose, saline, KCl, etiological and symptomatic drugs.

Discussions

Giardiasis is a cosmopolitan parasitic disease, endemic to tropical and subtropical areas, which can also occur in small family or collective groups with precarious hygiene, or as hydric epidemics after consumption of contaminated water. Sporadic cases of lambliasis may occur in children or adults that travel in highly endemic areas (Mexico, South America, Asia, Africa, Russia, etc.), or with a high risk of contamination (Vesy 1999, 846).

Giardia lamblia was experimentally proven to be transmitted by the ingestion of at least 10 cysts. This theory explains the high possibility of contamination between family members, in communities of adults or children with low hygiene or food conditions. The digestive pathway for transmission in food or water poisoning was also studied and documented. Beside these, the sexual pathway was also proposed in male homosexual collectives (Muhsen 2012, S273).

"*Giardia* is a flagellated, binucleated protozoan, discovered by Dutch microscopist Antonie Van Leeuwenhoek in 1681" (Syed 2003, 453), and "*Giardia* may exist in two distinct forms—cyst and trophozoite" (Hawrelak 2003, 129). Cysts, the infectious stages of the parasite, are continuously or intermittently eliminated with faeces. In the outer environment, mainly in moisture or water, they can reside for a long time. They are also resilient to chemicals used to disinfect water for public consumption, where they may survive for nearly two months (Vernile 2009, 203). Their relatively high resilience as cysts favours their ubiquitous presence in the environment. However, they are easily destroyed at temperatures of 65 degrees Celsius.

The main transmission pathway is faecal-oral. People are infected by ingesting mature cysts directly from other people, or indirectly from contaminated food or water. The incubation time is between 6 and 15 days, when the first symptoms may occur (Hawrelak 2003, 129). Direct transmission from one person to another may occur in precarious hygiene conditions, crowded places, promiscuity, dirty hands, especially in child communities, chronic disease hospitals, psychiatric hospitals, orphanages, asylums, etc.

Various species of fly can play a role in passively moving the cysts, as well as wind, which may carry parasitic cysts to the surface of food products, especially in the warm seasons. Faecal-oral transmission is considered by most specialists as the main way to disseminate the infection by *Giardia lamblia* (Rópolo 2010, 2019).

The infection with *Giardia lamblia* may cause clinically manifested conditions, evolving with acute diarrhoea as the dominant symptom, accompanied by stomach pain, nausea, vomiting, flatulence, anorexia and fever. Some of the patients develop a self-limited form of the disease, with spontaneous remission (Muhsen 2012, S273). Most patients have persisting diarrhoea, with malabsorption and weight loss for several weeks, requiring etiologic treatment to achieve a clinical and parasitological cure. We noted that in our group of patients the objective changes were less severe, and clinical features were dominated by digestive symptoms, followed by extra-digestive symptoms (neuropsychiatric and allergic).

The universally spread giardiasis involves both sexes and all ages, thus receptivity to *Giardia lamblia* is general.

Infection with *Giardia intestinalis* may evolve without clinical changes, in asymptomatic carriers, that eliminate cysts for more than six months, or may cause digestive and general symptoms with varying intensity and duration, depending on the massiveness of the infection and on the general and local resilience of the host organism. The disease is frequently diagnosed after visiting chronic patients from day centres or nursing homes (Vesy 1999, 846). The results we obtained demonstrate that 50% of the institutionalized elderly patients had acute diarrhoea, 8.82% had chronic diarrhoea, and 17.64% had alternating diarrhoea and constipation.

Positive diagnosis is established by demonstrating *Giardia* cysts in faeces, and more rarely trophozoides in diarrheic stools, duodenal fluid or jejunal biopsy. Cysts are continuously eliminated in the acute stage of the disease, and afterwards, as the infection tends to become chronic, they are intermittently eliminated, leading to false negative results. This is the reason why coproparasitologic exams should be repeated after 5–7 days in suspicious cases. Coproparasitologic examination is usually sufficient for the positive diagnosis of giardiasis. Cysts may be demonstrated microscopically with the direct examination of faeces, in physiological solution or Lugol solution, or by concentration techniques. Fresh stool examination for cysts is performed on specimens coloured with iodide or after conservation with formalin 10% or polyvinyl alcohol, and then coloured with trachoma solution or ferric haematoxylin solution.

Modern methods are based on demonstrating the *Giardia lamblia* antibody in stool samples. Some authors state that the gold standard for the diagnosis of giardiasis is the combined use of microscopy and ELISA (Vesy 1999, 847). Jejunal intestinal biopsy is an exceptional method in the diagnosis of lambliasis though it seems to be the most reliable since it allows both identification of the parasites in the mucus, at the surface of intestinal mucous or in intervilositary spaces, and histological assessment of the jejuna mucous. In general, intestinal biopsy is recommended in most cases to exclude another cause of malabsorption. The presence of the antibodies anti-*Giardia* may indicate either a previous infection or a current one, while identification of antigens of *Giardia* in faecal material point to an active infection. The specificity of the methods of identification of antigens has been improved by using monocolonal antibodies detrimental to the use of specific *Giardia* antigens such as glycoproteins in the cystic wall with a molecular weight of 31 and 65 kD using the ELISA technique and counterimmunoelectropheresis (Julio 2012, 5). Even with all the progress in deciphering the mechanisms and physiopathologic processes, giardiasis continues to be a worldwide health issue.

Conclusions

Knowing the prevalence of digestive lambliasis in institutionalized elderly patients allows the enforcing of specific prophylactic and treatment measures to lower the incidence of this parasitosis in elderly communities.

Measures will have to be taken to establish individual, collective and food hygiene rules in all nursing homes, together with improving medical and housing conditions.

Programs need to be implemented in elderly nursing homes concerning digestive infections with oral transmission, which would help to improve individual and food hygiene conditions for all the members of these communities.

References

Hanevik, K., Dizdar, Vernesa, Langeland, Nina & Hausken, T. (2009). Development of functional gastrointestinal disorders after *Giardia lamblia* infection. *BMC Gastroenterology 9 (1)*: 1-5.

Hawrelak, J. (2003). Giardiasis: pathophysiology and management. *Altern Med Rev. 8(2)*: 129-42.

Júlio, C., Vilares, A., Olaestro, M., Ferreira, I., Gomes, S., Monteiro, L., Nunes, B., Tenreiro, R. & Angelo, H. (2012). Prevalence and risk factors for *Giardia duodenalis* infection among children: a case study in Portugal. *Parasit Vectors 5*: 22.

Muhsen, K. & Levine, M. M. (2012). A Systematic Review and Meta-analysis of the Association Between Giardia lamblia and Endemic Pediatric Diarrhoea in Developing Countries. *Clinical Infectious Diseases 55 (suppl 4)*: S271-S93.

Rópolo, A. A. S. & Touz, M. M. C. (2010). A Lesson in Survival by *Giardia lamblia. The Scientific World Journal 10*: 2019-2031.

Syed, A. Alia & Hill, D. R. (2003). *Giardia intestinalis*. *Current Opinion in Infectious Diseases 16*: 453-460.

Vernile, A., Nabi, A. Q., Bonadonna, L. & Briancesco, Massa S. (2009). Occurrence of *Giardia* and *Cryptosporidium* in Italian water supplies. *Environ Monit Assess 152*: 203-207.

Vesy, C. J. & Peterson, W. L. (1999). Review article: the management of Giardiasis. *Alimentary Pharmacology & Therapeutics 13 (7)*: 843-50.

IMPACT ASSESSMENT OF PARTICULATE MATTER EMISSIONS AND RESPIRATORY PATHOLOGY IN RESIDENTS LIVING CLOSE TO LIGNITE QUARRIES

DELIA NICA-BADEA

Introduction

The exploitation of coal, and thermal power plants using coal as fuel, can influence the environment, sometimes leading to the affectation of ecological balance in the areas where they are located, representing a complex impact on all environmental factors in their neighbouring area of atmosphere, water, soil, flora and fauna, food and passenger compartment. The operating, transportation and storage of coal create a significant amount of fine particulate matter suspended in the air. Suspended particles are a complex mixture of organic and inorganic compounds which negatively affect the human body (Gautam et al. 2012; Epstein et al. 2011).

The potential toxic appreciation of suspended particulates depends on the following factors: size, composition and origin; the process of particle formation; the defence mechanism of the respiratory system and the breathing pattern (Câra et al. 2007; Nica-Badea, Popa & Gămăneci 2011). Particles and liquid and gaseous materials that are absorbed and taken together with the particles, if they are toxic, may contribute to organ damage, such as the kidneys and the liver. There are a variety of methods for measuring various fractions of suspended particulates in the air, with different meanings for the health status.

Recent studies are focused on the health effects caused by short-term, acute exposures to suspended particles. Both types of studies have shown that chronic and acute exposures alike cause significant negative effects on human health, although the toxicological mechanisms for these effects are lesser known (Simendić & Nebojša 2012; Kumar & Sharma 2012; Pinheiro et al. 2007; Schwella 2001). The particulate matter is introduced into the body by inhalation and deposited in the human respiratory system; therefore, exposure to air pollution can lead to significant health problems because pollutants in the air inevitably affect the respiratory tract (see Figure 3-2 below). The emitted particulate matter in the atmosphere leads to increasing mortality and morbidity through respiratory disease. Generally, the effects on health display features associated with the thoracic (PM10) and/or breathable fraction (PM2.5) (Neamţu, Moldoveanu & Staicu 2009).

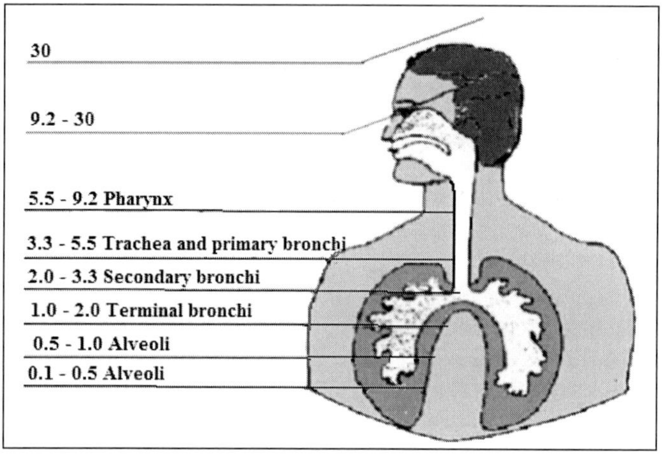

Figure 3-2. Depth of penetration of particles in the body, depending on their size (μm) (Simendić & Nebojša 2012)

Particulates cause health effects through three mechanisms: direct mechanical type (irritating) on the upper respiratory tract; systemic toxic effects; and an indirect effect through the carriage of substances having a secondary effect (Hendryx & Ahern 2008; Kumar & Sharma 2012; Schwella 2001). The concentration of particles in suspension and sediment is associated with a wide range of adverse effects on health, including acute or chronic respiratory ailments, increasing the number of hospitalisations for diseases of the respiratory tract (Atkinson et al. 2001).

Some studies have found that residents of coal mining communities have a 70% increased risk of developing kidney disease, a 64% increased risk of developing chronic obstructive pulmonary disease, and a 30% risk of hypertension (Hendryx & Ahern 2008). Other studies revealed a dose-response-like result where communities residing in areas of high mining activity presented the highest all-cause mortality rates and the highest chronic heart, respiratory and kidney disease rates, areas of low coal mining activity had lower rates, and areas with no coal mining had lower rates still (Hendryx 2009). One study demonstrated that residents of coal mining communities reported significantly fewer healthy days both mentally and physically, and rated their overall health to be poorer than residents of non-mining communities (Zulling & Hendryx 2010).

A high incidence of respiratory diseases in children under the influence of anthropogenic pollutants was observed, in particular of the suspended particles PM10, PM2.5 emitted mainly by exploitation and processing of mineral resources, which have adverse effects even at concentrations below accepted standards. Acute pulmonary first or second in childhood may be due to microbial or viral infection or may have an allergic etiopathogenesis element, such as an air pollutant, as the main factor (Batesen & Schwartz 2008; Câra et al. 2007; Gouveia & Fletcher 2000; Hruba et al. 2001; Neamţu, Moldoveanu & Staicu 2009).

The pointer in PM10 Gorj County exceeded the limit values of daily and annual viewing of the population protection caused by the combined intake of several sources: residential heating in the cold season, exploitations and quarry activity, and burning fossil fuels for producing electricity (Gorj Environment Protection Agency 2010; Neamţu, Moldoveanu & Staicu 2009).

Materials and Methods

This study is based on analysis of the dust level in the functional area and the respiratory pathology of lignite among communities as a result of the evaluation of statistical data concerning medical reporting, risk associated with exposure to hazardous substances, and marine risk on the health condition of the population. In this context, the study proposes the correlation structure between ground level concentrations of particulates and pathological respiratory hazards in the coal quarries.

The Roşiuţa Quarry is part of Mine Motru subunit of the National Society of Lignite Oltenia. Coal deposit, which serves the quarry, is located in this area in Roşia near the national road DN 67 connecting the cities of Târgu-Jiu, Motru and Drobeta Turnu-Severin. The population of research localities have 1,987 inhabitants, divided as: Roşiuţa (746), Ploştina (1160) and Lupoaia (81). These villages belong to Motru City.

The study uses the database Mining Exploitation Quarries Motru to achieve a correlation structure between level concentrations of particulates and pathological respiratory hazards in the coal quarry areas (Roşiuţa, Gorj County) made in selecting and developing stages and methods of the study (Gautam et al. 2012; Neamţu, Moldoveanu & Staicu 2009; Savu Iliescu & Curcă 2009).

Monitoring of particulate sedimentable matter in the functional area near the coal deposit was made through the automatic method (nefelometric) and the reference method (gravimetric). Risk assessment on the health of the population in the area of influence of the coal quarries was to analyze statistical data addressing the correlation of risk factors associated with exposure to hazardous substances by case-control studies of the relationship type Odds Ratio (OR) and statistical analysis in linear regression model univariate and multivariate relationship between exposure and potential effects on population health stations.

The application of statistical analysis of the correlation in the regression model can provide data on the relationship between the frequency of being taken ill and the concentration of certain dangerous substances. Therefore, two scenarios were tested: scenario A (worst case) for the expected concentrations in emissions based on the permitted limits; and scenario B (real case) for concentration estimated in emissions based on limits measured in the coal deposit area. Each dangerous substance in the database has been associated with specific related afflictions.

For the coding and grouping of chronic pathology by category of disease, we used the ICD-10 classification (International Classification of Diseases). The frequency of being taken ill based on the current frequency of being taken ill in the study area, and forecast values for dangerous substances and environmental factors as a result of the functioning of the objective of the review, were made in the Microsoft Excel and Statistics Trial programmes.

Results

Average concentration of particulate matter

Published statistical data of the concentrations of suspended particulates nationwide for the years 2008–2009 reflects an overrun of the maximum permitted concentration, the annual average for PM10, in the counties of Gorj, Dolj, Vâlcea and Mehedinţi, known for lignite thermoelectric exploitation and processing (see Figure 3-3 below). Monitoring the air quality network in the area of analysis (coal quarry range) for Total Suspended Particles (TSP) pollutant covered the 7 points of the sampling, the sample being disposed in 7 houses of the village of Roşiuţa (P1-P7). For sedimentary powder, the air quality monitoring network in Roşiuţa quarry encompassed 8 sample points, samples arranged in 7 residences in

Roşiuţa village and one in Lupoaia Railway Station (P1-P8). The average concentration of particulate matter (samples of short duration at 30 minutes), and the average concentration of sedimentary powder measured monthly in 2009 in all sampling points, in comparison with the Maximum Admitted Concentration (M.A.C), are shown in Table 3-9 below.

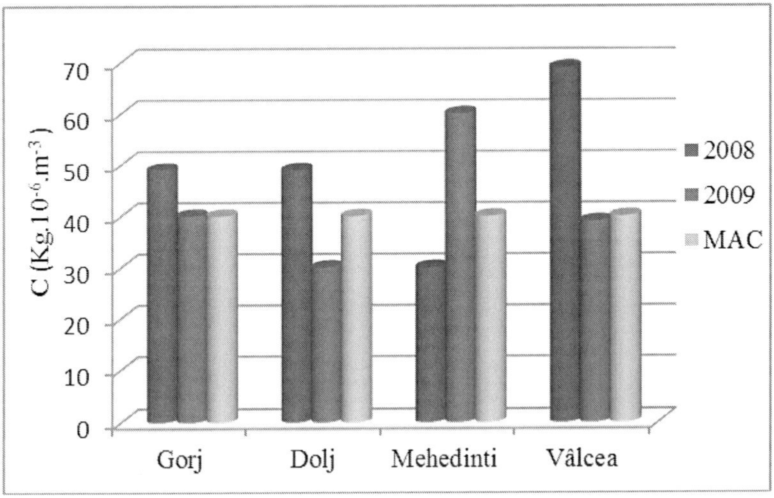

Figure 3-3. Annual average concentration of PM10 in districts adjacent to the quarry of lignite (Neamţu, Moldoveanu & Staicu 2009)

Table 3-9. The average concentration in sedimentable and suspensor dust (quarry areal)

	PM sedimentable		PM suspended	
Sample points	C. average monthly Kg.10^{-3}.m^{-2}	M.A .C. Kg.10^{-3}.m^{-2}	C. average 30 min Kg.10^{-6}.m^{-3}	M.A .C Kg.10^{-6}.m^{-3}
P1	26.42	17	0.029	0.50
P2	28.16	17	0.068	0.50
P3	18.33	17	0.064	0.50
P4	30.37	17	0.11	0.50
P5	26.73	17	0.076	0.50
P6	11.45	17	0.091	0.50
P7	18.73	17	0.029	0.50
P8	7.60	17	-	-

Data Addressability

The study of addressability at the municipal Motru hospital comprised 165 subjects, ages ranging between 1 and 87, 51.68% women and 48.32% men.

Statistical data on the average age: median age (51.51761), standard deviation (21.15986), kurtosis (-1.04548), skewness (-0.04886), minimum (0.980986), maximum (87.06117), count (165). The distribution map, in absolute terms, of the cases of chronic diseases in the period 2007–2009, emphasizes the following order related to: pathology of pregnancy (46); chronic respiratory (38); cardiovascular (23); asthma (10); strokes (10), osteoarticular (10); ulcerous diseases (9); kidney diseases (6); malignant (5); dermatitis (3); haematological (3); diabetes mellitus (2). The data distribution statistics for addressability (diagnostic), for asthma and chronic respiratory disorders, in the area of influence of the coal has the following: Roşiuţa (asthma: 30%, chronic respiratory: 31%); Ploştina (asthma: 60%, chronic respiratory: 65%); Lupoaia (asthma: 10%, chronic respiratory: 4%). The addressability, for asthma and chronic respiratory disorders, in the area of influence of the coal store is shown in Figure 3-4 below.

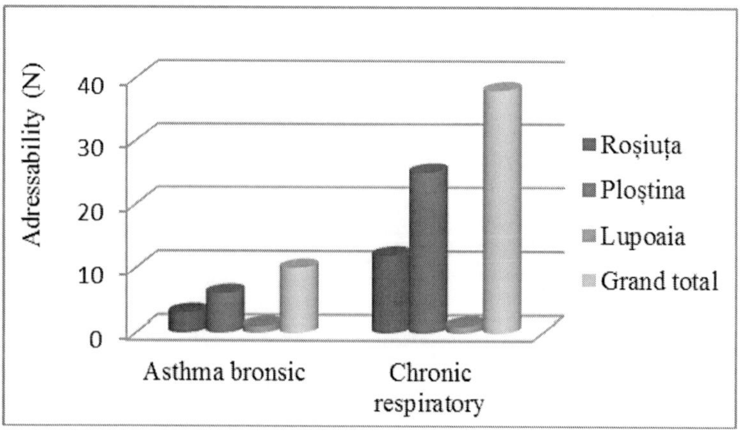

Figure 3-4. Addressability residents for asthma bronchic and chronic respiratory diseases (diagnostic) (2007–2009)

Assessment of the Risk Associated with Exposure to Hazardous Substances

Studies of case-control Odds Ratio (OR) were carried out to compare the risk of developing a chronic pathology over time, studied in Roşiuţa, the nearest area by the point of interest compared to the other areas in the analysis zone (see Table 3-10 below).

Table 3-10. Data correlation risk factors of pathological respiratory effects Odds ratio (OR)

Variables	Bronchic asthma			Chronic respiratory disease		
	Effect present (cases) Zone 1	Effect absent (control) Zone 2	Total	Effect present (cases) Zone 1	Effect absent (control) Zone 2	Total
Present risk factor	3	7	10	12	26	38
Absent risk factor	743	1234	1977	743	1234	1977
Odds value	0.004	0.0056	0.71	0.0016	0.020	0.76

Zone 1: Roşiuţa, Zone 2: Ploştina and Lupoaia; CI 95%, p=0.05

The Odds Ratio represents a way to compare if the probability of apparition of a given event is the same for the two groups. The Confidence Interval is a range of values with a high probability of containing the parameter that was estimated (CI 95%). Calculation of the relative risk estimate presents the following values: for asthma (odds cases: 0.0040, odds witnesses: 0.0056, OR: 0.71) and chronic respiratory (odds cases: 0.01, odds witnesses: 0.020, OR: 0.76).

The risk assessment on the health condition of the population is reflected in the statistical analysis in linear regression model univariate and multivariate of the relationship between exposure and the potential effects on the population's health stations. The tables below contain statistical processing on the relationship between frequency of illness and the concentration of certain hazardous substances (concentrations provided by Mining Exploitation Quarries Motru and Environmental Protection Agency Mehedinti). For each dangerous substance (those provided) diseases that are specifically related to them have been associated.

Discussion

The concentration of suspended particulate matter (PM) for 2009 has not exceeded the allowable average values (0.50 Kg.10^{-6}. m^{-3}) for an averaging time of 30 minutes. The maximum permissible level of sedimentary powder concentration level (17 $Kg.10^{-3}.\ m^{-2}$) for 2009 was exceeded 1.1–1.7 times in the area of influence of coal (see Table 3-9 above).

There were overruns in 2010 regarding the maximum permitted by the sedimentary powders concentration (65.31 $kg.10^{-3}.\ m^{-2}$ maximum monthly), the average trend being a subunit fraction. In 2010 the measuring was focused on lead, arsenic, cadmium and nickel by the atomic absorption spectroscopy method of particulate matter PM fraction collected on filters in automatic air quality monitoring. There was no exceeded limit value prescribed regarding annual target values, in accordance with the rules in force. Loading the atmosphere with particles in suspension is due to the warehouse of the coal quarry and intense traffic, resulting from the increase in the number of vehicles and the fact that the warehouse is located next to the national road DN 67. Studies have found that out of the total sedimentary dust, the lignite powder represents 72.85%–81.73% and the rest is road dust.

A baseline study on the health status (baseline) refers only to chronic pathology investigated distribution without trace association between health status and concentration of certain hazardous substances in environmental factors (currently and in the future). Meanwhile, the baseline survey of health provides an overview of chronic pathology in the areas influencing objective investigation.

Addressability for asthma and chronic respiratory diseases in the villages of the area influenced by the coal deposit is in descending order: Ploştina, Roşiuţa and Lupoaia (see Figure 3-4 above). The impact assessment of respiratory pathologies through statistical data relevant to the entire area, according to the availability to the practitioner, holds a pathology related to pregnancy, followed by chronic respiratory diseases. For respiratory pathology, availability for asthma and chronic respiratory diseases reflect a distribution which is inversely proportional to the distance from the object of study.

To assess the risk associated with exposure to hazardous substances, an Odds Ratio (OR) was done to compare the risk of developing a chronic pathology over time in Roşiuţa, the area nearest the lens of interest compared to the other areas in the analysis. The odds ratio represents a way to compare if the probability of apparition of a given event is the same for the two groups (see Table 3-10 above).

For asthma, "the report chances" of developing a disease are less in the case of comparisons between the exposed area (Roșiuta—Zone 1) and unexposed areas (Ploştina and Lupoaia—Zone 2), being present and statistically significant for each of the areas compared. Thus, exposure rate cases are less than the exposure rate to witnesses.

In terms of exposure as a risk factor, in this case exposure reduces the risk of disease (OR <1 safety factor).

In terms of overall chronic respiratory diseases, "the report opportunities" to develop a chronic respiratory disease are less in the case of Zone 1 comparisons, statistical significance, if OR subunit, not present in either case. If we compare Zone 1 and Zone 2, the OR was less than unity, without being statistically significant. A nil OR value reflects the fact that the chances of developing a chronic respiratory disease are higher in residents of Zone 2, compared with those living in Zone 1, and this is statistically insignificant.

Scenario A (worst case) refers to estimated concentrations-based emission limits in permits-coal deposit. Statistical models (scenario A-worst case) showed no statistically significant correlation between the frequency of chronic bronchitis and maximum permitted levels of PM10 respirable particles in the air (an annual average, and average maximum daily and hourly rates for the year under review). Regarding emphysema and chronic obstructive pulmonary disease, the frequency of cases is significantly correlated with the maximum permitted levels of PM10 respirable particles in the air (the average daily and hourly maximum value for the year under review). Frequency of asthma in the study area was not significantly correlated with the maximum permitted levels of respirable particles PM10 (annual average, average daily maximum hourly value for the year under review). On interstitial lung disease, the frequency of cases is significantly correlated with the maximum permitted levels of PM10 respirable particles in the air (the average daily and hourly maximum values for the year under review).

Scenario B (real case) analyzes the estimated emission concentration limits based on measured existing deposits. Relation to the linear regression model in the frequency of chronic respiratory disease (chronic bronchitis, emphysema, chronic obstructive broncho-pneumopathy, asthma, interstitial lung disease) with measured levels of PM in suspension (as daily average and hourly maximum values for the year under review) did not give a statistically significant correlation between the frequency of chronic respiratory diseases analyzed and measured levels of PM. What differentiates Scenario A from Scenario B, in terms of modelling adverse effects in relation to exposure to pollutants, is that there is no correlation between the frequency of obstructive pulmonary emphysema and chronic exposure to PM in suspension (either average daily and hourly values) in the multivariate model or the univariate models, and the frequency of these diseases is not correlated with exposure to PM in suspension. The frequency of occurrence of these diseases should be viewed in the context of the above scenario A.

Conclusion

The main health effects caused by exposure to particulate matter are respiratory and heart diseases. Pollutants leading to the emergence of both diseases that have specific chronic and acute respiratory pathologies are those that correspond to at least PM10 thoracic faction and/or respirable PM 2.5, NOx, SO_2 and ozone. Acute pulmonary diseases may be due to microbial or viral infections, or may be known as the main factor allergic etiopathogenesis element can be an air pollutant. Nationwide and local areas and periods in excess of the maximum permitted dust levels are in direct correlation with incidence pathologies. State level of respiratory diseases among communities in mining areas, as a main etiopathogenic element regarding maximum levels of respirable particulate matter PM, are the result of the effects of anthropogenic factors of synergism and operating environment, transport, storage and processing of the lower heating of coal. The results show that there is a cause-effect association between levels of particulate matter in the atmosphere caused by the operation, transport, storage and processing of lignite and the respiratory diseases of people in the surrounding areas. It is imperative for the health of residents' research mechanisms, extent and consequences of the effects of the coal quarries.

References

Atkinson, R.W., Anderson, H. R., Sunyer, J., Ayres, J., Baccini, M., Vonk, J. M., Boumghar, A., Forastiere, F., Forsberg, B., Touloumi, G., Schwartz, J. & Katsouyanni, K. (2001). Acute effects of particulate air pollution on respiratory admissions. *American Journal of Respiratory and Critical Care Medicine 164 (10)*: 1860-1866.

Batesen, T. F. & Schwartz, J. (2008). Children's response to air pollutants. *Journal of toxicology and environmental health 71 (3)*: 238-243.

Câra, A. C., Frank, B., Geert-Jan, D. & Sârzea, V. (2007). Polluting the atmosphere, a risk factor for respiratory diseases in children. *Romanian Medical Magazine 14 (1)*: 11-15.

Epstein, P. R., Buonocore, J. J., Eckerle, K., Hendryx, M., Benjamin, M. S., Heinberg, R., Clapp, R. W., May, B., reinhart, N. L., Ahern, M. M., Doshi, S. K. & Glustrom, L. (2011). Full cost accounting for the life cycle of coal. *Annals of the New York Academy of Sciences 1219(1)*: 73-98.

Gautam, A., Kumar, A. P. & Kumar, B. P. (2012). Opencast mines: a subject to major concern for human health. *International Research Journal of Geology and Mining 2 (2)*: 25-31.

Gorj Environment Protection Agency. (2010). *Annual Report on State of the Environment in Romania for 2010*. Online: http://www.anpm.ro/Mediu/raport_privind_starea_mediului_in_romania15.

Gouveia, N. & Fletcher, T. (2000). Respiratory diseases in children and outdoor air pollution in Sao Paolo, Brasil: a time series analysis. *Occupational and Environmental Medicine 57 (7)*: 477-483.

Hendryx, M. & Ahern, M. M. (2008). Relations between health indicators and residential proximity all coal mining in West Virginia. *American Journal of Public Health 98 (4)*: 669-671.

Hendryx, M. (2009). Mortality from heart, respiratory, and kidney disease in coal mining areas of Appalachia. *International Archives of Occupational and Environmental Health 82 (2)*: 243-249.

Hruba, F., Fabianova, E., Koppova, K. & Vandenberg, J. J. (2001). Childhood respiratory symptoms, hospital admission, and long term exposure to airborne particulate matter. *Journal of Exposure Analysis and Environmental Epidemiology 11(1)*: 33-40.

Kumar, H. & Sharma, A. (2012). Air Pollution: A Fatal Attack on Cardio-Respiratory System. *British Journal Human Social Science 3 (2)*: 2048-1268.

Neamţu, A., Moldoveanu, A. M. & Staicu, C. (2009). Impact assessment of public health atmospheric pollutants irritating and carcinogens. *The National program to monitor the determinants of life and work environment*. Bucharest: National Centre for Monitoring of Risks in the Community. 15-19.

Nica-Badea, D., Popa, R. G. & Gămăneci, Gh. (2011). Impact of environmental risk factors anthropogenic respiratory pathology. *Proceedings of the National Symposium with International participation, 2nd edition, Respiratory pathology in current medical practice, Aprilie 28-29, 2011, Târgu-Jiu*: 59-60.

Pinheiro, T., Bugalho de Almeida, A., Monteiro, P., Alvarez, E., Moniz, D., Alves, L. C. & Freitas, M. C. (2007). Particulate matter and health—from air to human lungs. *Assessment of levels and "health-effects" of airborne particulate matter in mining, metal refining and metal working industries using nuclear and related analytical techniques*. Vienna: IAEA TECDOC-1576. 165-182.

Savu, D. V., Iliescu, Fl. & Curcă, I. (2009). Study to assess the risk of an impact on health of residents in the area deposit of coal quarry Roşiuţa. *Raport Contract 621/s/2009 SNLO beneficiary, Târgu Jiu, EMC Motru*: 70-104.

Schwella, D. (2001). Air pollution and health in urban areas. *Revue Environ Health 5*: *13-42.*

Simendić, B. & Nebojša, J. (2012). Monitoring of suspended and respirable particulate matter in the city of Novi Sad. *Monitoring and expertise in safety engineering 2 (3)*: 8-17.

Zulling, K. J. & Hendryx, M. A. (2010). A comparative analysis of health-related quality of life for residents of U.S. counties with and without coal mining. *Public Health Reports 125 (4)*: 548-555.

SOCIAL AND MEDICAL PERCEPTIONS OF CHRONIC ALCOHOL CONSUMPTION IN PATIENTS WITH LIVER DISEASE

ELENA TOADER

Introduction

The amplitude of negative health effects of chronic alcohol consumption turn this phenomenon into a social interest issue beyond the boundaries of the strictly scientific medical awareness. Currently, the comprehensive approach on chronic alcohol consumption entails the attention granted to the relevance of the medical impact (health impact), the social representation manner, the economic and professional impact, the necessity of health policy intervention and the ethical and cultural significance of the phenomenon. An important role in the formation of the representations on chronic alcohol consumption is played by the social context in which the information on the contents and dynamics of the phenomenon circulates. Because of its magnitude, alcohol consumption is perceived in the Romanian environment as a phenomenon with a complex social impact, defined by the increasing number of consumers and illnesses caused, but also by the illicit actions it generates (Room, Babor & Rehm 2005). Taking into account the fact that the consumers' tendency is increasing and the age of the public consumer is decreasing, both current status and predictable tendencies turn chronic alcohol consumption into a phenomenon with inferences within the social, professional and especially family environments. In this chapter we focus on the interface between the healthcare system and social environment and describe the representation of the phenomenon through the summarization of the medical, economic and political implications, followed by an exploration of the perceptions of patients diagnosed with chronic liver disease caused by chronic alcohol consumption. There are too few studies in the literature that investigate the social representation of alcohol consumption in patients with liver disease or that integrate this phenomenon into the management of the alcoholic liver disease beyond the strictly etiologic ascertainment. We believe that the approach of this issue in a mixed framework (medical and social) is a novel characteristic which introduces the implications of chronic alcohol consumption regarding the predictability of negative outcomes on the individual as a patient from a complex medical, social, economic and familial perspective, as well as from the point of view of the political strategies, into the debate.

Chronic alcohol consumption and impact on health. The association between alcohol consumption and health problems has been known for a long time, but the complex and multidimensional nature of this relationship was mostly revealed in the last thirty years. Scientific research in this area advanced steadily, bringing substantial contributions for a better understanding of the medical implications of alcohol consumption as well as for the elaboration of strategies and measures for the prevention and treatment of the diseases caused by it. Numerous papers remark on the fact that alcohol influences health through an increase in mortality and the risk of serious disease, while the epidemiologic descriptors reveal the proportion and dimension of invalidity caused by alcohol consumption, proven to be the main cause of over 60 diseases and a major cause for social issues, traumas and early death (Room, Babor & Rehm 2005). In the European Union, 7.4% of disease or early death cases are caused by alcohol abuse (Rehm et al. 2010), an aspect which causes a legitimate concern regarding chronic consumption. According to OECD statistics, in Romania the yearly alcohol consumption is as high as 12.7 litres by inhabitant and medical issues caused by this behaviour are recorded in over 50% of cases (Khazan 2012). Liver damage caused by alcohol consumption is reported as one of the most frequent negative consequences on health under its various forms (hepatitis, cirrhosis and liver cancer) in the context of simple or occasional consumption, but also in the pattern of exaggerated and, especially, irregular alcohol consumption, recognized as a major factor (Cox & Klinger 1988). Research results for the threshold of noxious alcohol consumption (defined as a drinking pattern which causes deterioration of health, either physical—e.g. cirrhosis or mental condition—or depression secondary to alcohol consumption) seem to agree that almost no consumption pattern is completely without risks. Consumers should be aware that the benefits deriving from drinking must be put into balance with a series of risks for their health, because liver, heart, lung or neuropsychic disease could develop in any individual within this context (Murray 2013).

Moreover, the extent of the issues generated by alcohol consumption goes from the individual (patient) level to the social space of the community to which they belong, a feature which imposes that the adequate medical approach be completed by a basic intervention in the healthcare for the general population or at risk from this disease.

Interventions in primary healthcare. Although medical research, correlated in the last few decades with social and economic interventions, brought remarkable contributions to the establishment of the dimension of chronic alcohol consumption, systematic comments indicate the focus of the main healthcare system on the curative aim, leaving little room for prevention interventions for this unhealthy behaviour. The practice confirms that primary healthcare does not use instruments for the identification of the individuals at risk of chronic alcohol consumption, and the management of the patient with alcohol-generated illnesses (e.g. liver disease) does not comprise a distinct component directly addressing alcohol consumption. Doctors and mainly general practitioners believe that general screening for health issues caused by alcohol does not represent an adequate strategy, although they do feel compelled to intervene when confronted with various pathologic conditions generated by it (Lid & Mlaterud 2012). The fact that there are too few doctors who initiate conversations with the patient about alcohol consumption denotes an attitude and a behaviour which mirrors the belief that their main mission is to treat the problems generated by alcohol (diseases) and not preventing alcohol consumption (Nygaard & Aasland 2011).

Political and economic interventions. The negative effects of alcohol consumption (over 195,000 deaths every year in the EU and an economic cost of 125 billion Euros) justify the concerns in the healthcare policies area (Anderson & Baumberg 2006). As a response to the increasing recognition of the negative impact on health of alcohol consumption, the European Commission offered support to member states through the adoption of the first strategy (October 2006) regarding the approach and combat modalities against the negative effects of alcohol. From the five objectives of the strategy we mention the control of the damages associated with respect to health, social and economic impact, as well as the organization of sensitivization activities. The application of these strategic objectives implies the integration of the policies from the entire union, which may have an impact on the efforts undertaken in this area, materialized in actions of identification of the best practices within the framework of a forum on alcohol and health. Moreover, in this forum clear commitments will be made by experts from the organizations taking part, representatives of the member states and European healthcare institutions for the investigation of several specific subjects such as the relationship between alcohol consumption and inequities in healthcare area, or the elaboration of scientific notifications for the modulation of alcohol consumption in risk groups (with an emphasis on young people).

The **Economic impact of alcohol consumption**, assessed through direct and indirect costs, represents another domain of interest where multiple pieces of information circulate which can be used as logistical support for strategies and politics in this territory. The economic effects of alcohol abuse are as damaging to the community as the effect on the health of the individual, for involvement is equally important for the patient, family and community. Alcohol abuse contributes to an increase in healthcare costs, estimated to be twice as high for the families with one member with an alcohol issue, while almost half of the emergency requests are related to alcohol (Chan & Harris 2007). However, society tends to treat the medical and social consequences of alcohol abuse rather than its causes. Although the evidence, the experience and the arguments in favour of the negative impact of chronic alcohol consumption are bigger than those for any other drug, it seems that the public and medical concern for the prevention and treatment of this addiction are lower than for other major diseases or other drug abuse (Burke 1988). The solutions to these problems could be successfully found through the analysis of the determining factors that trigger this addiction, which should be, in turn, integrated into sectorial policies and strategies.

In the second part of this chapter we focus on the exploration of the social influences and medical perceptions of patients with chronic liver disease about chronic alcohol consumption.

Our main objectives are regarding the medical perceptions of alcohol consumption of patients with chronic liver disease explored within the framework of the causality relationship between alcohol and liver disease and of the management of the patient with alcoholic liver disease, as well as the social perception of alcohol consumption, with an emphasis on the social environment's attempts to identify the motivations for alcohol consumption but also the manner in which it influences the life of the individual.

Methods

We selected patients with chronic liver disease (N=254) and a history of alcohol consumption, confirmed through their biomedical records or an AUDIT questionnaire. The relationship between the medical and social representation of chronic alcohol consumption was assessed through a questionnaire oriented on two directions: the relationship with the healthcare system and the requirements of the social environment, with separate sections attributed to the interest and information in the medical, social and cultural context associated with the phenomenon (causality relationship with alcohol-disease, motivation to drink, access to healthcare, the healthcare system in Romania, benefits, risks and costs of alcohol consumption, influences and impact on behaviour and management of the patient with alcoholic liver disease) and even details about the phenomenon exposed freely as answers to certain questions. The information was gathered into a database for statistical processing and for the descriptive report (Table 3-11). Taking into account the role assigned to alcohol consumption within the context of the personal history of the responders and their experiences inside the healthcare system, we take advantage of the data obtained from these patients. We chose to perform this study at the Gastroenterology and Hepatology Institute in Iasi because here the chronic liver disease can be diagnosed and medically overseen according to standards for both inpatients and outpatients.

Results

In 89% of cases the medical perception of responders on alcohol consumption was focused on healthcare strategies with a curative purpose (therapeutic interventions). The evidence of these observations is yielded by the fact that, although they admit the negative health impact of alcohol consumption, only 35% accept the fact that their current disease (liver disease) is correlated with the custom to drink and only 11% are following a maintenance therapy. In 67% of the cases the motivations for alcohol consumption were correlated with a context of influences originating in the social and familial relationships, but also with the quality of financial resources. A cultural representation of alcohol consumption was noted in 15% of the patients. The relevance of the social environment requirements with respect to alcohol consumption resulted in the association of certain details of the answers to the questions where 81% of the patients appreciated, with (self)-criticism, the influences and impacts on health. However, 19% of the patients do not yet have a clearly defined point of view, or exhibit denial of the direct relationship between alcohol and liver disease.

Table 3-11. Medical and social perception of alcohol consumption in patients with chronic liver disease

1. Medical perception of alcohol consumption—relationship with healthcare system	
Question	***Answer (254 patients with chronic alcoholic liver disease)***
(a) causality relationship between alcohol and disease	
Generally speaking, do you believe alcohol consumption to be a health concern?	50% Yes 35% Yes (when you go beyond the limit) 15% It depends on the individual
Do you believe that your current disease (liver disease) has a connection with your custom to drink?	35% Yes 20% Possibly 50% No
(b) management of the patient with alcoholic liver disease	
How often do you come to the doctor (hospital) for health issues presented after alcohol consumption?	89% for medical care with curative purpose (therapeutic intervention) 11% for maintenance and prevention therapy
Have you assessed the benefits, risks and costs of alcohol consumption?	76% No 14% I didn't think about it 10% did not answer
What are the reasons for your drinking?	67%—relationships and familial or social issues, quality of financial resources 15% No reason 18% did not answer
2. Social perception of alcohol consumption—social environment requirements	
How do you regard the influence of alcohol consumption in your life?	72% Normal (I do not drink until intoxication) 18% *I abuse it*
In what circumstances do you drink?	15% cultural representation (events, parties, funerals, etc.)
Is alcohol a solution to your problems? (justification of alcohol consumption)	69% Yes (I had some problems, there are many difficulties) 17% I don't know 14% did not answer
What are the influences and impact of alcohol consumption on your behaviour?	81% I abuse it 10% I am not aware 9% did not answer
Will you be willing to give up alcohol consumption?	50% Yes 25% I should do it 12% I'll think about it 13% did not answer

Discussion

(1) Medical perception of patients with chronic liver disease on alcohol consumption. The data confirmed that the perceptions of the patients regarding alcohol consumption and causality of liver disease derive from the value attached to health and from the representations founded on the educational and cultural context of the community and social space they belong to. The manner in which the patient processes the medical information concerning alcohol consumption determines the significance of the details memorized during contact with the healthcare system. The fact that most patients (89%) appeal to the health system for curative care implies the interest and importance given to the information of a medical nature about the current (liver) disease but not to alcohol consumption, because only 11% come back to the system to continue the program of healthcare and prevent relapse. Other distinctions that are worth mentioning are for the patients (a great number) with experience in the healthcare system who do not realize the financial and economic implications deriving from alcohol consumption (excessive consumption of healthcare, consumption of resources from the National Fund of Social Security, less resources for the contributors), which result from repeated hospitalizations in various situations, and some even criticise their importance. The facilitation of the access to healthcare and its quality are the foundation for an anticipative socialization of a permissive relationship with the healthcare system in Romania where they benefit from free assistance focused on the effect (assistance with the disease) but not the cause (alcohol consumption, prevention, strategies), as can be observed from the obtained data (89% curative healthcare versus 11% maintenance and prevention).

(2) Motivation of alcohol consumption. Alcohol consumption—a solution to certain issues—this is the perception of the patients on the reasons to drink alcohol with the signification of the "over demand" by various relational components in the family, workplace, and the financial and professional nature of their job or society. For the patient, alcohol consumption is perceived as a way to neutralise certain tensions, dissatisfactions or disappointments. Moreover, while the emphasis is placed on the relationship with demand formulated as distinct (e.g. familial issues) or cumulative motivations (family, job, money), the patient does not perceive the social significance of the "costs" for the healthcare system due to the fact that they are free and supported by the state budget. Furthermore, many of those assisted by the system do not have health insurance and do not contribute to the social security fund, but benefit, without restrictions, from healthcare services, generating through the excessive consumption of resources an inversion in the ratio between beneficiaries and contributors and hence inequities in the healthcare system (Ladar 2006).

(3) Family and alcohol consumption is an extremely important area of debate through the key position and the double role played by the family in the management and therapy plan of the patient with liver disease, and also in the range of motivations for alcohol consumption. For most of the patients, family occupies a central place in the representation of the phenomenon, negatively associated with a series of issues that become a source for an explanation of the disease (e.g. the departure of a family member for work abroad). A positive association for the role of the family is identified in the context of the relationship as "therapeutic control" of the patient, through active involvement, to ensure the conformation to the treatment and prevention of the relapse.

(4) Alcohol and social networking. For the patient with chronic liver disease, alcohol consumption is responsible for certain forms of social networking. Acceptance, adherence and integration in communities where chronic alcohol consumption is practiced develops a motivational dimension with double signification: cultural, respecting traditions for alcohol consumption to certain events (weddings, christenings, funerals, etc.), and a personal one of denial or lack of acceptance of a negative impact of drinking on health or as direct cause of liver disease (Larsen et al. 2009). In the personal case, this last argument occurs frequently as dissociated, the individual (patient) adopting a distinct attitude towards the disease (liver damage) and another towards alcohol consumption, apparently without a direct causality relationship, although most patients indicate problems as the common denominator for both situations (disease and addiction).

Limits of the Study

Although the results of this exploratory study cannot be generalized they may indicate a general tendency in the medical and social representations of patients with chronic liver disease developed after alcohol consumption. For the cultural differences in the perception of alcohol consumption we did not focus on the different interpretation of alcohol consumption in women and men, because we believe that in order to explore the significations in this direction adjusted methods are necessary, with semi-structured interviews. Another limit of the study is related to a series of affirmations incompletely justified and uncorrelated with the biomedical findings and AUDIT questionnaire, as well as under certain optimal answers. For these reasons, we associated freely expressed opinions with answers to certain questions, developing the interpretation of the results obtained in patients with a high AUDIT score, where the intervention for alcohol consumption is mandatory. Interestingly, great differences were not recorded between patients with low and high AUDIT scores, a possible explanation being the modality of cultural representation of alcohol consumption supported by certain similarities in motivations and the rural origin of both categories of patients.

Conclusions

We can state that the problems generated by chronic alcohol consumption continue to represent a major challenge for science, public health and society, as long as an approach for the general population seems to be ignored by the public healthcare system in favour of an individually oriented strategy that tends to be more palliative than preventive. The results from this exploratory study on the social and medical perception of chronic alcohol consumption in patients with liver disease can also be recorded in this direction. Thus, the medical and social representations of the alcohol consumption of the responders are structured on a series of themes interconnected which reveal the domination of the curative medical approach offered by the legal framework of the healthcare system, and less the preventive, addressed to the causal factor of alcohol consumption. From the point of view of the social representation of alcohol consumption, we can notice the interference of the multifactorial motivational range and the cultural component, an association which in most cases generates new negative stimuli that support this addiction. Consequently, the evaluation of the motivational structure for chronic alcohol consumption through the identification of the medical, social, cultural, financial, etc. influences can bring about initiatives, actions and reactions in the healthcare domain able to generate changes in the management of the patient with alcoholic liver disease beyond the strictly curative interventions.

References

Anderson, P. & Baumberg, B. (2006). *Alcohol in Europe. A Public Health Perspective. A Report for the European Commission*. Online: http://ec.europa.eu/health/ph_determinants/life_style/alcohol/documents/alcohol_europe.pdf.

Burke, T. R. (1988). The Economic Impact of Alcohol Abuse and Alcoholism. *Public Health Reports 103*: 564-568.

Chan, S. & Harris, J. (2007). *Nuffield Council on Bioethics: An ethical review of publications*. Online: http://www.nuffieldbioethics.org/.

Cox, M. W. & Klinger, E. (1988). A Motivational Model of Alcohol Use. *Journal of Abnormal Psychology 97 (2)*: 168-180.

Khazan, O. (2012). Which Europeans are fattest, laziest and drink most, in charts. Online: http://www.washingtonpost.com/blogs/worldviews/wp/2012/12/04/which-europeans-are-fattest-laziest-and-drink-most-in-charts/.

Ladar, C. (2006). Finanțarea sectorului sanitar II. Hazardul moral o problemă comună a finanțării bazate pe asigurările de sănătate [Financing the Health Sector II. Moral Hazard: A Common Issue of Financing Based on Health Insurance]. *The Journal of the Faculty of Economics—Economic Science Series XV (II)*: 316-320.

Larsen, H., Engels, R. C., Granic, I. & Overbeek, G. (2009). An Experimental Study on Imitation of Alcohol Consumption in Same-Sex Dyads. *Alcohol & Alcoholism 44 (3)*: 250–255.

Lid, T. G. & Mlaterud, K. (2012). General practitioners' strategies to identify alcohol problems: A focus group study. *Scandinavian Journal of Primary Health Care 30*: 64-69.

Murray, E. (2013). *Screening and brief intervention for alcohol use disorders in primary care*. Online: http://dx.doi.org/10.1136/bmj.e8706.

Nygaard, P. & Aasland, O. G. (2011). Barriers to implementing screening and brief interventions in general practice: Findings from a qualitative study in Norway. *Alcohol 46*: 52-60.

Rehm, J., Baliunas, D., Borges, G. L., Graham, K., Irving, H., Kehoe, T., Parry, C. D., Patra, J., Popova, S., Poznyak, V., Roerecke, M., Room, R., Samokhvalov, A. V. & Taylor, B. (2010). The relation between different dimensions of alcohol consumption and burden of disease: An overview. *Addiction 105 (5)*: 817843.

Room, R., Babor, T. & Rehm, J. (2005). Alcohol and public health. *Lancet 365*: 519-530.

ASYLUM: POLITICAL PERSECUTION AND EXTRADITION OF CRIMINALS

CLAUDIA-LIVIA ANDRIȚOI AND ADINA-IULIA NICOLAE

Introduction

The actuality of the asylum concept derives from the massive displacement of people, especially in the twentieth and twenty-first centuries, to our country due to the level of eco-socio-political development of the area in which it is located, and military conflicts and economic crises that have disrupted people, triggering massive displacement, which give a special importance to the institution of political asylum and extradition, being differentiated by the various forms of migration and refugee institution. Political asylum does not have a distinct approach, and it is not regulated as a stand-alone institution.

The notion of asylum is rooted in the ancient Greek *asilon* which is a form of the adjective *asyl* ("inviolable"). In the terminology of the Latin origin term *asylum* (asylum), it means "it cannot be pursued" or "could not be arrested," "protection against persecution," "retreat" or "safe," "location of the protection, shelter, refuge" (Potîngă & Costachi 2003, 48).

Some authors believe that the concept of asylum is "granted by a state law establishing its territory of persons wanted in their country for political or religious reasons" (Breban 1991, 84), or "by a state grant to setting within pursued or persons in their country."

Methods

The interpretative method. From the analysis of the definition of asylum in international and regional documents on the matter, it appears that the notion of refugee is treated, not asylum. Even where reference is made to the concept of asylum, the approach is similar to that referred to above and which states: "the right to grant protection to people who for reasons of race, religion, nationality, membership of a particular social group or political opinion are outside the country of his nationality and is unable or, owing to such fear, unwilling to protect this country" (Delcea 2002, 36).

The structuralist method. The Declaration on Territorial Asylum adopted by the UN General Assembly on February 14, 1967 separately analyzed the issue of asylum, being the only document tackling asylum internationally.

In the period after the Second World War, states have avoided a precise definition of the concept and its coverage of international agreements, for the following reasons:

- The economic situation after the war
- The emergence of barriers separating areas of interest
- The demonstration of superiority of one system over another
- A still confused situation of the attitude to be adopted by the states that still have a large number of colonies
- Visible revival of national consciousness of the third world countries.

The current attitude has the following reasons:

- developed countries changed in restrictive asylum policies, under pressure from the recession and not least because of nationalist and xenophobic movements.
- Ideological and political, internationally determined debates on human rights have diminished since 1989, and asylum has ceased to be used as evidence of the superiority of capitalism over communism.
- The former communist countries opposing asylum before the 1989 codification of ideological considerations are not currently interested in any of the coding because many are part of the "*cordon sanitaire*" protection of Europe, or transit countries located in the vicinity and generating asylum seekers.
- European countries as a whole are concerned with solving the current and future problems of integration, where no shelter is at the forefront, but it remains only to prove the continuity of the European humanitarian spirit and adjust the controlled immigration, including the police.
- Afro-Asian countries, and Central and South America, are fearful that after encoding asylum the burden will be passed to protect them while the international aid received is insufficient to help them cope with dignity (Delcea 2002, 36).

The epistemological method. South-American countries managed to achieve an acceptable encoding with clearer rules which will ensure the implementation of the Universal Declaration of Human Rights, art. 14. Thus, even if it precedes the Universal Declaration, the Convention on Political Asylum signed at Montevideo on December 26, 1933 at the Seventh International Conference of American States, defines the institution of political asylum as a "humanitarian institution."

Later, American states, backed by the Convention on Territorial Asylum signed in Caracas on March 28, 1954, showed that political asylum is a right of the state and that the exercise of this right does not cause the dissatisfaction of another state. In the Convention on Diplomatic Asylum, signed in Caracas on March 28, 1954 at the Tenth Inter-American Conference, art. 2 stressed that "every state has the right to grant asylum, but is not obliged to do so or to state the reasons for refusal to grant."

South American States come to the treaty on Political Asylum and Refugees, signed at Montevideo on April 8, 1939 and note that "asylum may be granted irrespective of nationality, and without prejudice to the rights and protection obligations accruing to the state to which the refugees belong, the State granting asylum is therefore obliged to admit refugees on its territory, unless they are not allowed entry into another state." Major progress can be seen through this treaty, in that it requires signatory states to admit refugees' access in certain exceptional situations, unlike the previous rules that left this to the discretion of the states.

The basic document through which the Central and South American states address the concept of asylum is the Convention on Asylum signed at Havana on February 2, 1928, where signatory states points out in art. 2 that by removing the context it "will be respected as a humanitarian law or by tolerating established usage, conventions or laws of the country as granted." Norms in Africa mainly emphasize the definition of a refugee and do not give due consideration to the asylum or asylum seeker. It is marginal, but in the second article asylum is defined in the Organization of African Unity Convention on the specific aspects of refugee problems in Africa, adopted in Addis Ababa on October 9, 1969, which states in paragraph 2 that: "The granting of asylum to refugees is a peaceful and humanitarian act and shall not be regarded as an unfriendly act by another Member State."

The same kind of approach and content meet the principles relating to the treatment of refugees adopted by the Afro-Asian Advisory Board from Bangkok 1966, which in art. III, § 1, shows that "a state has the sovereign right to grant or to deny asylum on its territory to a refugee," but paragraph 4 points out that the refusal situation "would be to ensure that asylum provisionally in such circumstances as it deems appropriate and will ensure the person can search and risk asylum in another country." As we have seen from the contents of the above, we can conclude, by avoiding a clear definition of political asylum in most areas, refugee problems have been tolerated.

Another feature is that the developing countries have shown a greater interest in finding the most appropriate instruments to address, but so far have not effectively resolved the problem. The developed countries and those of the former socialist bloc present a serious approach to the problem by sidestepping a precise formulation of the concept of political asylum and asylum in general, which would generate obligations and economic and social consequences. As we have pointed out how the problem is treated internationally and regionally, it is necessary to clarify that we cannot develop the proposed theme without performing the relevant national legislation. In this sense the Constitution shows that: "The right to asylum shall be granted and withdrawn under the law, respecting treaties and international conventions" (Mihăilă & Andrițoi 2009, 35).

Such a formulation was intended to remove what "is essentially a right belonging to foreigners and stateless persons," and "is hosting the protection that the state confers upon them." The comments made on this by Ion Muraru, one of the main editors of the text of the Constitution of Romania, are characterised by the following key features:

- Recognition of the right to asylum is made as a fundamental right
- It fixes the legislature and shall establish by law the cases and conditions in which asylum is granted or withdrawn
- Asylum should be granted or withdrawn in accordance with treaties and conventions to which the State is party.

Thus, we can clearly observe the fact that the constitution has highlighted the right of the individual and not the state, and is obviously granted in accordance with the interests of the state, with its internal regulations and with international or regional norms, to which our country is a party.

After the constitution defined the framework for addressing political asylum in general and in particular, the GO No. 102 of August 31, 2000 on the status of refugees in Romania, approved by Law no. 323 of 27.06.2001, amended and supplemented by GO No. 13 of January 1, 2002, subsequently approved by Law no. 264 of May 15, 2002 and amended by O.U.G. No. 76 of August 28, 2003, proceed directly to the concept of refugee treatment, avoiding asylum (Iancu 2002, 56, 76–78).

Discussions and Results

Can we appreciate that these rules were a diffusion of the term asylum at refugee status, and that it would mean the same thing or that there is an omission in this regard? We appreciate that, in the above-mentioned legal acts, there was a sense of strict interpretation in the Convention on the Status of Refugees, made at Geneva on July 28, 1951 and the Protocol on the Status of Refugees, adopted on November 18, 1967, therein analyzing the obligations of states in light of the Universal Declaration of Human Rights which did not lead to diverging views regarding the definition of asylum seekers. The politically preferred analysis and definition of the term refugee operating throughout the two acts somehow tried to cover aspects that characterize only asylum, but not defining it.

However, we must note that the two concepts have pronounced similarities but also differences that prevent any confusion between them. The following similarities can be extracted from the content:

- Both can be granted only to foreigners persecuted for various reasons
- Both are forms of humanitarian protection
- Providing both asylum and refugee status, the competence of the receiving state, by virtue of its sovereignty
- The rights the two groups receive are similar, with some nuances.

as well as the following differences:

- Preceding asylum is the status of refugee
- Asylum is regulated by the international or regional standards (unfortunately they do not provide any rigorous definition) rather than the national
- Refugee protection is involved immediately (temporarily) while the final status involves asylum
- Refugee status can be recognized, even if the person is granted asylum
- Rights and obligations of the two categories of persons holding different rights
- Procedures for two different forms of protection, and hence that the provisions relating to withdrawal, termination or cancellation of refugee status cannot be found for the right of asylum (for which I have not made a detailed approach)
- The beneficiary of the right to asylum cannot be extradited, unlike the beneficiary of refugee status, which can expel limited circumstances prescribed by law

- Refugee application is state law
- The granting of refugee protection status produces no legal effect on family members.

However, we must note that the two concepts have pronounced differences that prevent any confusion between them. The following similarities can be extracted:

- Both can be granted only to foreigners persecuted for various reasons
- Both are forms of humanitarian protection
- Providing both asylum and refugee status confers competence to the receiving state, by virtue of its sovereignty
- The rights the two groups receive are similar, with some nuances

as well as the following differences:

- Preceding asylum status is the refugee status
- Asylum is regulated in the international or regional standards (unfortunately they do not provide any rigorous definition) rather than the national
- Refugee protection is involved immediately (and temporarily) while the final status involves asylum
- Refugee status can be recognized, even if the person is granted asylum
- The rights and obligations of the two categories of persons holding different rights
- Procedures for two different forms of protection, and hence the provisions relating to withdrawal, termination or cancellation of refugee status, cannot be found for the right of asylum (for which I have not made a detailed approach)
- The beneficiary of the right to asylum cannot be extradited, unlike the beneficiary of refugee status, who can be expelled under limited circumstances prescribed by law
- Refugee application is state law
- The granting of refugee protection produces no legal effect on family members
- For the asylum status an intern or international protection institution right doesn't exist (Iancu 2002, 56, 76–78).

Conclusions and Proposals

Regarding political asylum, many different themes can be approached providing a detailed analysis of numerous issues including the relation between the institution of asylum and extradition of criminals, which is a current concern for many organisations or international forums because many criminals have penetrated the great wave of refugees and applicants for asylum status, persons who, in order to avoid application of the law to acts committed in their home state, turn to the institution of asylum to avoid the consequences of their application.

With regards to the extradited persons requesting refugee status or asylum, who have committed a crime in their home state, there is a general international consensus, but different interpretations appear regarding the extradition of persons who were granted a form of protection and there is an attitude of rejection of the extradition request, especially from EU member states and those who adhere to this structure. When it comes to the extradition of a person to their home in which they have been sentenced to death, all these and other procedural issues are aimed at cooperation with international criminal legalities, especially concerning the institution of extradition addressed by the treaty signed by the UN General Assembly and adopted by resolution on September 16, 1990 nr.45/116, and the European Convention on Extradition, adopted in Paris on December 13, 1957, supplemented by additional protocols in Strasbourg on October 15, 1975 and March 17, 1990, with changes to the convention implementing the Schengen Agreement of June 19, 1990.

Since UNO documents do not recognize general rules on the subject, there are some opposing views of how to address this organization, especially on the issue of extradition of asylum seekers who have committed crimes in their country of origin. Due to the small number of acceding countries relying heavily on European devices, it is generally accepted in this field that there is a large consensus of countries in the region. First, we would like to highlight the need for such rules which constitute the general rules for other bilateral documents developed and adopted in the matter of extradition.

In order to support the development and adoption of general international norms almost all assessments of theorists in this field come into play, showing that "extradition as a rule is due to the bilateral effect" (Wallace 1997, 120), and that "there is no obligation to extradite in the absence an international treaty."

In support of the necessity of such treatment, some authors argue that "extradition treaties don't release either of the two parties involved from their obligations" (Ibid.), which ensures the fulfilment of international justice.

Also, in addition to the opinions of more or less authorized specialists, they find it useful to recall the definition adopted at the Tenth Congress of the Association of Penal Law, which leads to the same conclusion, namely the need for international regulation and cooperation, without which the extension of internal international enforcement can take effect. The definition adopted by these states is that: "Extradition is an act of interstate judicial assistance in criminal matters, of the transfer of an individual prosecuted or convicted by the judicial sovereignty of a State by the other State" (Oxford Advanced Learner Dictionary of Current English 1974, 125).

Extradition can only be the result of international cooperation, for the administration of justice to individuals who are no longer in the judicial sovereignty of the state through another state or international organizations, occurring as a result of developments at the institutional level.

Although in the past asylum was considered as a barrier to universal repression against offenders and that, while deeply evolved as a tool for the effective protection of persons undergoing persecution of any kind, especially the political and religious ideas (an area in which there is a similar development period of inquisition), there is no way that in the shadow of this institution, particularly generous and with a deep humanitarian character, that common criminals can hide (Mihăilă & Andriţoi 2009, 105)

We estimate that the conditions for extradition could be as follows:

- Facts need to be established regarding the law of the requesting Party and of the requested Party (subject to extradition including deeds amnesty in the requested State, Article 62, sentence 2, the Schengen Agreement, June 14, 1985).
- Punishment should be the deprivation of liberty or a detention order of imprisonment for a minimum of one year in the first case, or at least four months in the second.
- If the extradition concerns more facts and not all meet the above conditions, it is granted and they may remove an express renunciation of the specialty rule (Article 66, sentence 2 of the Schengen Agreement, June 6, 1985).
- Laws of signatory states may express reservation in respect of the above conditions (which was expressed even by Law 302/04 on judicial cooperation in criminal matters, which increases the length of

sentences and security measures for necessary extradition to two years). This measure becomes operational only after notifying the Secretary general of the Council of Europe.

- Reciprocity can occur in offenses excluded from the scope of the convention (exclusion can operate only under certain procedural conditions).
- Extradition shall not be granted for political offenses, even if it is apparently presented as a common law offence.
- An exception to this requirement.
- Attempt on the life of a Head of State or a member of their family.
- Crimes against humanity under the Convention on the Prevention and Punishment of the Crime of Genocide, adopted by the UN on December 9, 1948.
- Crimes concerning the treatment of prisoners of war and protection of civilian persons in times of war from the wording of the Geneva Conventions of 1849 and 1949.
- Any violations of the laws or customs of war in the Convention on the treatment of prisoners of war and the Convention on the Protection of Civilian Persons in times of war of the 1949 Geneva Convention.
- No extradition granted for military offences.
- There is an obligation to extradite their nationals, with the obligation to submit their judicial authority, competent in handling the case concerning the offence for which extradition was requested.
- Extradition may be refused for an offence committed partly or wholly in the requested state.
- Extradition may be refused if the person sought is extraditable for the same offence or was tried and finally convicted for the same offense by the competent authorities of the requested party.
- Extradition will not be granted when the person has been tried and convicted by a state.
- Acquittal.
- Punishment or security measures have been fully executed.
- They have been the subject of a pardon or amnesty.
- No penalty or sanction has been imposed.
- Extradition may be refused where the requested state considers that the trial in absentia of the person in question did not satisfy the minimum rights of recognized defence. It can still be given if we receive an assurance considered sufficient regarding a new procedure of the court.
- Extradition shall not be granted if the prescription is fulfilled regarding prosecution or punishment under the law of a party.
- Extradition will not be granted when the person has a death sentence.

As we can see from the study of the conditions listed, some of them are mandatory, preventing extradition, while for others the requested party leaves the decision to extradition operability

We proceeded to such a group as we consider that it satisfies a greater need to focus their rapid extraction conditions to be fulfilled on a first legal examination (Mihăilă, Stan & Suciu 2006, 89).

Of those recorded above, the attitude that states do nothing to create the necessary legal framework in the exercise of their sovereign right to join, fully or with reservations, the agreed upon framework to govern the institution of extradition, has inspired many other related rules ensuring their necessary basis for legislation and bilateral treaties, which correspond to finally achieving the essential objective of carrying out justice. It can, however, be put in another way.

References

Breban, V. (1991). *Dicţionar general al limbii române* [General Dictionary of the Romanian Language 1]. Bucureşti Ed. Enciclopedică—Ed. RAI.

Delcea, M. (2002). *Protecţia juridică a refugiaţilor în dreptul internaţional* [The legal protection of refugees in international law]. Timişoara: Presa Universitară Română.

Iancu, Gh. (2002). *Dreptul de Azil. Privire comparativă cu statutul juridic al refugiatului* [Asylum: Comparative legal status of refugee]. Bucureşti: ALL Beck.

Mihăilă, M. & Andriţoi, C. (2009). *Protecţia juridică a drepturilor omului* [Human rights and anti-discrimination strategies]. Reşiţa: Eftimie Murgu.

Mihăilă, M., Stan, D. & Suciu, C. (2006). *Tratat de drept internaţional public* [Public international law treaty 3]. Bucureşti: BREN-V.I.S.PRINT.

Oxford Advanced Learner Dictionary of Current English. (1974). Oxford: Oxford University Press.

Potîngă, A. & Costachi, Gh. (2003). *Asigurarea drepturilor omului în lume* [Ensuring human rights worldwide]. Chişinău: Epigraf.

Wallace, M. M. R. (1997). *International Law*. London: Sweet and Maxwell.

CONTRIBUTORS

Felicia ANDRIONI is currently a Lecturer at the University of Petroşani, Romania. She holds a BA in Social Work from the "Babeş-Bolyai" University of Cluj-Napoca, Romania, an MA in International Project Management from the National School of Political Science and Administration of Bucharest, Romania, and a PhD in Sociology from the "Babeş-Bolyai" University of Cluj-Napoca. Her main areas of interest include social sciences, education sciences, culture, and environmental protection. She has published widely in the field of social work.

Claudia-Livia ANDRIŢOI is currently an Associate Professor at the "Eftimie Murgu" University of Reşiţa, Romania. She holds a BA in Law from the "Iosif Constantin Drăgan" European University of Lugoj, Romania, an MA in Public Administration Management from the "Eftimie Murgu" University of Reşiţa, and a PhD in Theory of General Law from the West University of Timişoara, Romania. Her main research interests are human rights, international law and general theory general law. She has authored *Principiile interpretării în ordinea juridică pozitivă* (The principles of interpretation in positive judicial order) (2010), *Investigarea interpretării juridice şi a rezultatului acesteia prin intermediul semanticii şi hermeneuticii juridice* (The investigation of judicial interpretation and its result through judicial semantics and hermeneutics) (2010), co-authored *Protecţia juridică a drepturilor omului* (Judicial protection of human rights) (2009), *Drepturile omului şi strategii antidiscriminatorii* (Human rights and anti-discriminator strategies) (2009), and *Dreptul internaţional public între întrebări şi răspunsuri* (Public international law in questions and answers) (2009).

Ştefania BEJAN is currently a Lecturer at the "Alexandru Ioan Cuza" University of Iaşi, Romania. She holds a BA in Philosophy and an MA in Social Anthropology and Ethnology from the "Alexandru Ioan Cuza" University of Iaşi, and a PhD in Philosophy from the same University. Her main research interests are mass communication, public relations, and political theories. She has authored *Discursul Educaţiei* (The Discourse of Education) (2003) and edited *Caiete Sociologice* (Sociological Review) (2003-2008).

Cornel CONSTANTINESCU is currently an Associate Professor at the University of Piteşti, Romania. He holds a BA and a PhD in Sociology from the University of Bucharest, Romania. His main research interests are sociology of education, sociological research methodology, and Romanian sociology history. He has authored *Arhivarea şi analiza secundară a cercetării sociologice* (Archiving and secondary analysis of sociological research) (2003) and *Metode şi tehnici de cercetare sociologică – caiet de aplicaţii practice* (Sociological Research Methods and Techniques: Book of Practical Applications) (2007), and co-authored *Sociologia educaţiei* (Sociology of Education) (1998), *Industrialisation, developpement economique et social, La zone Argeş—Piteşti, Roumanie* (Industrialisation, Economic and Social Development: The Argeş—Piteşti Area, Romania) (2006), and *La protection du maillon le plus faible* (Protection of the Feablest Chain Loop) (2009).

Maria CONSTANTINESCU is currently a Professor at the University of Piteşti, Romania. She holds a BA in Psychology and a PhD in Sociology from the University of Bucharest, Romania. Her main research interests are human development, psycho and family assistance, child protection, human resource management, migration of parents and children personality. She has authored *Competenţa socială şi competenţa profesională* (Social Competence and Professional Competence) (2004), *Sociologia familiei. Aspecte teoretice şi aplicaţii practice* (Sociology of Family. Theoretical and Practical Applications) (2004), *Familia românească între tradiţie şi modernitate* (Romanian Family Tradition and Modernity) (2008), *Dezvoltare umană şi asistenţă socială* (Human Development and Social Work) (2008), and edited *La protection du maillon le plus faible Social Work in European Context* (2008), (Protection of the Feablest Chain Loop) (2009), and *Boosting Entrepreneurship Tools for Migrants* (2012).

Dănuţ-Ioan CRAŞOVAN is currently a Lecturer at the "Mihai Eminescu" University of Timişoara, Romania. He holds a BA in Psychology and an MA in Clinical Psychology from the West University of Timişoara, and a PhD in Psychology from the University of Bucharest, Romania. His main research interests are psychological defence mechanisms and coping mechanisms in various medical conditions. He has authored Concepte fundamentale, tehnici şi teorii de *Metodologia de cercetare în psihologie* (Fundamental Concepts, Techniques and Theories of Research Methodology in Psychology) (2009), *Bazele testarii psihologice* (Bases of

Psychological Testing) (2011), and *Bazele psihologiei experimentale* (Bases of Experimental Psychology) (2011).

Dan-Ioan DASCĂLU is currently an Assistant Professor at the "Ştefan cel Mare" University of Suceava, Romania. He holds a BA in Sociology from the University of Bucharest, Romania, and a PhD in Psychology from the "Alexandru Ioan Cuza" University of Iaşi, Romania. His main research interests are totalitarianism, political social psychology and the dimensions of contemporary individualism. He has authored *Comportamentul consumatorului* (Consumer behavior) (2002) and co-authored *Vilolenţa în sport* (Violence in sports) (2006).

Alin GAVRELIUC is currently a Professor at the West University of Timişoara, Romania. He holds a BA in Sociology and an MA in Political Sciences and Administration from the same University, a PhD in Social Psychology from the University of Bucharest, Romania, and a Habilitation in Psychology from the "Babeş-Bolyai" University of Cluj-Napoca, Romania. His main research interests are cross-cultural psychology, social psychology and ethno-psychology. He has authored *O călătorie alături de "celălalt". Studii de psihologie socială* (A journey next to the "other". Studies in social psychology) (2002), *Mentalitate şi societate. Cartografii ale imaginarului identitar din Banatul contemporan* (Mentality and society. A symbolic identitary maps from contemporary Banat) (2006), *Viaţa ca prilej. 101 oglinzi psihosociologice despre "ceea ce suntem"* (Life as a matter. One hundred one psycho-sociological mirrors about "what we are") (2008), *De la relaţiile interpersonale la comunicarea socială* (From interpersonal relationships to social communication) (2007), *Psihologie interculturală. Repere teoretice şi diagnoze româneşti* (Inter-cultural psychology: Theoretical framework and Romanian diagnosis) (2011), and *Româniile din România* (Romanias from Romania) (2011).

Dana GAVRELIUC is currently a Lecturer at the West University of Timişoara, Romania. She holds a BA in Psychology and an MA in Educational Sciences from the same University, and a PhD in Psychology from the "Babeş-Bolyai" University of Cluj-Napoca, Romania. Her main research interests are educational psychology, social psychology and cross-cultural psychology. She has authored *Caiet de practica pedagogica. Specializarea psihologic* (A Handbook of Pedagogical Practice. Psychology) (2010) and *Scoala si schimbare sociala* (School and social change) (2012).

Maria-Ana GEORGESCU is currently an Associate Professor at the “Petru Maior” University, Tîrgu Mureş, Romania. She holds a BA in Philosophy from the “Babeş-Bolyai” University, Cluj-Napoca, Romania, an MA in Management of International Relations and European Affairs from the “Petru Maior” University, Tîrgu Mureş, and a PhD in Sociology from the “Babeş-Bolyai” University, Cluj-Napoca. Her main research interests are socioeconomics, ethical dimension of business activities and public administration, entrepreneurial education, social management. She has authored *Educaţie şi mobilitate socială* (Education and Social Mobility) (1998), *Bazele microeconomiei* (Fundamentals of Microeconomics) (2003), *Sociologie* (Sociology) (2005), *Provocări socioeconomice* (Socioeconomics Challenges) (2005), and *Etica între teorie şi acţiune* (Ethics between Theory and Action) (2011).

Emilia HERMAN is currently an Associate Professor at the “Petru Maior” University of Târgu Mureş, Romania. She holds a BA in Economics from the same University and a PhD in Economics from the “Babeş-Bolyai” University of Cluj-Napoca, Romania. Her main research interests are labour market, entrepreneurial economy, and regional development. She has co-edited *Macroeconomie* (Macroeconomics) (2011).

Claudia-Anamaria IOV is currently a Research Assistant at the “Altiero Spinelli” Center for the Study of European Governance, “Babeş-Bolyai” University of Cluj-Napoca, Romania. She holds a BA in History and International Relations, an MA in International Relations and European Studies, and a PhD in International Relations and European Studies from the “Babeş-Bolyai” University of Cluj-Napoca, and a PhD in Geopolitics from the University Paris 8 Vincennes Saint-Denis of Paris, France. Her main research interests are inter-ethnic relations in South-Eastern Europe, migration as a security matter, ethnicity and intercultural dialog with emphasis on the Roma problem within EU. She has published widely in the field of sociology, security studies and international relations.

Amador JIMÉNEZ-GARRIDO is currently a PhD Candidate at the University of Jaen, Spain, and a Teacher for Denver Public Schools in Denver, CO, United States. He holds a BA in Education Sciences from the University of Jaen, and an MA in Applied Linguistics from the University of Granada, Spain. His main research interests are bilingualism, language learning strategies and lexicography. He has published widely in the field of linguistics.

Beniamin LUP is currently president of WorldTeach Association of Timişoara, Romania, and a lawyer with Advocates International, Fairfax, VA, USA. He holds a BA in Law and an MA in Criminal Justice from the from the West University of Timişoara. His main research interests are constitutional law, human rights and dignity, and criminal justice. He has published widely in the fields of law and human rights.

Ştefan-Sebastian MAFTEI is currently a Lecturer at the "Babeş-Bolyai" University of Cluj-Napoca, Romania. He holds a BA, an MA and a PhD in Philosophy from the "Babeş-Bolyai" University of Cluj-Napoca. His main research interests are philosophy of art, rhetoric, hermeneutics, and contemporary philosophy of culture. He has authored *Geniul artistic: Nietzsche şi problema creaţiei artistice. Între romantism şi avangarda germană* ("The Artistic Genius": Nietzsche and the Problem of Artistic Creation. Between German Romanticism and the German Avant-Garde) (2010).

Ramona MALIŢA is currently an Associate Professor at the West University of Timişoara, Romania. She holds a BA in Humanities Studies from the University of Oradea, Romania, an MA in Humanities Studies from the West University of Timisoara, and a PhD in Philology from the "Babeş-Bolyai" University of Cluj-Napoca, Romania. Her main research interests are French and Francophony Literature and traductology.

Mihai MAREŞ is currently an Associate Professor at the "Ion Ionescu de la Brad" University of Iași, Romania. He holds an MD and PhD in Microbiology from the "Gr. T. Popa" University of Medicine and Pharmacy of Iași. His main research interests are medical mycology and human reproduction, with research emphasis on new antimicrobial molecules and microbial induced infertility. He has edited *Chlamydia* (2012).

Iosif MARINCU is currently an Assistant Professor at the "Victor Babeş" University of Medicine and Pharmacy of Timişoara, Romania. He holds an MD, an MA in Social Medicine and Health Management, and a PhD in Medicine from the same University. His main research interests are viral hepatitis, HIV/AIDS infections, zoonoses, antibiotics therapy, trichinelosis, and pneumonia. He has authored *Diagnosticul infecţiei cu virusul hepatitic C* (Diagnosis of infection with hepatitis C virus) (2002) and co-authored *Răspunsul organismului la infecţii* (Body response to infection) (2001).

Marian MIHĂILĂ is currently a Professor at the "Eftimie Murgu" University of Reşiţa, Romania. He holds a BA in Law from the "Alexandru Ioan Cuza" Police Academy of Bucharest, Romania, an MA in Humanitarian international law from the University of Bucharest, and a PhD in International Law from the "Alexandru Ioan Cuza" Police Academy of Bucharest. His main research interests are public international law, protection of cultural property in international law and environmental law. He has authored *La protection des biens culturels dans le droit international* (The protection of cultural property in international law) (2003), *Tratat de drept internaţional II, III* (A Treatise of international law II, III) (2005, 2006), *Elemente de drept internaţional public* (Elements of public international law) (2009) and co-authored *Tratat de drept internaţional I* (Treatise of international law I) (2004) and *Drept instituţional comunitar* (Community international law) (2007).

Ioana-Delia NADOLU is currently a Lecturer at the West University of Timişoara, Romania. She holds a BA and an MA in Sociology from the same University, and a PhD in Sociology from the "Babeş-Bolyai" University of Cluj-Napoca, Romania. Her main research interests are social anthropology, anthropology of the space, mythology, and rural-urban sociology. She has authored *Socio-antropologia spaţiului* (Socioanthropology of the Space) (2004).

Delia NICA-BADEA is currently a Lecturer at the "Constantin Brâncuşi" University of Târgu-Jiu, Romania. She holds a BA in Chemistry and Physics from the University of Bucharest, Romania, an MA in Nutrition Sciences from the "Babeş- Bolyai" University of Cluj-Napoca, Romania, and a PhD in Chemistry from the University of Bucharest. Her main research interests are interdisciplinary approach of chemistry and physics applied, instrumental analytical chemistry, nutrition science, nutrition - doping in sports, preservation and restoration of cultural property, biochemistry and biophysics exercise, health education and social medicine. She has authored *Noţiuni fundamentale de biofizică cu aplicabilitate medicală* (Fundamentals of Biophysics Applied in Medicine) (2014), *Controlul principiilor active din produse alimentare excitante* (Control of Active Principles of Food Stimulants) (2011), *Ştiinţele nutriţiei I* (Nutrition Sciences 1) (2011), *Controlul agenţilor dopanţi în sport* (Control of Dopant Agents in sport (2009), *Elemente de chimia conservării, restaurării operelor de artă* (Elements of Artefact Conservation and Restoration Chemistry) (2009), and co-authored

Cromatografia pe strat subţire. Analiza produselor alimentare (TLC: Analysis of the food (2005).

Adina-Iulia NICOLAE is currently an Assistant at the "Eftimie Murgu" University of Reşiţa, Romania. She holds a BA in Public Administration and an MA in Management of Public Institutions from the same University, and a PhD in Economy from the "Lucian Blaga" University of Sibiu, Romania. Her main research interests are human rights, international law, community law, migration and its economic impact. She has published widely in the field of sociology.

Laura-Cristina OPRICĂ is currently a Teacher at the School of Orodel, Dolj County, Romania. She holds a BA in English Language and Literature and an MA in Anglo-American Studies from the University of Craiova, Romania. Her main research interests are in the field of theories, methods and techniques used in language learning and in educational technology and other resources used in learning a foreign language.

Eufrasio PÉREZ-NAVÍO is currently a Professor at the University of Jaen, Spain. He holds a BA in Psychology-Pedagogy from the same University, an MA in Quality of Higher Education from the University of Las Palmas, Gran Canaria, Spain, and a PhD in Educational Sciences from the National Distance Education University of Madrid, Spain. His main research interests are teacher training, ICT in Education and Innovation in Education. He has authored *Procesos y Contextos Educativos* (Educational Processes and Contexts) (2009) and *Sociedad, Familia y Educacion* (Society, Family and Education) (2010).

Lavinia-Elisabeta POPP is a Lecturer at the "Eftimie Murgu" University of Reşiţa, Romania. She holds a BA in Social Work and an MA in Educational Marketing Management from the same university, and an MA in Family and Family Resource Management and a PhD in Sociology from the "Alexandru Ioan Cuza" University of Iaşi, Romania. Her main areas of interest are social work and sociology. She has published widely in the field of social work.

Silvia RUSU is currently a Research Assistant at the West University of Timişoara, Romania, and a PhD Candidate in Psychology at the "Alexandru Ioan Cuza" University of Iaşi, Romania. She holds a BA in Psychology and an MA in Organizational Psychology from the same University. Her main research interests are implicit measures of personality and their ability to predict behavior, Semantic Misattribution Procedure as an implicit measure of self-concept, changing implicit cognition in smokers using evaluative conditioning procedures, and work—life balance. She has co-authored *Metode implicite de investigare a personalităţii* (Implicit measures in personality assessment) (2011).

Roxana SÂRBU is currently a Psychologist at the Career Counselling Centre of the West University of Timişoara, Romania. She holds a BA in Psychology and an MA in Organizational and Leadership Psychology from the same University. Her main research interests are career information, career counseling, career development and personality psychology. She has co-authored *Abilităţi psihologice – un ghid pentru profesori şi studenţi* (Psychological Skills: A guide for Teachers and Students) (2009).

Daniela SPÎNU is currently a PhD Candidate at the University of Bucharest and at the Ecole doctorale francophone en sciences socials of Bucharest, Romania. She holds a BA in Political Science and an MA in European and Romanian Politics from the University of Bucharest. Her main research interests are internal migration during the Soviet period, Romanian emigration and the security issues related to international migration. She has published widely in the field of social scienes.

Elena TOADER is currently an Associate Professor at the "Gr. T. Popa" University of Medicine and Pharmacy of Iaşi, Romania. She holds a BA in Law from the "Alexandru Ioan Cuza" University of Iaşi, an MA in Health Management from the National School of Public Health and Health Management, Bucharest, Romania and a PhD in Medicine from the "Gr. T. Popa" University of Medicine and Pharmacy, Iaşi. Her main research interest is clinical research. She has authored *Rectocolita Ulcerohemoragica* (Ulcerative colitis) (2011) and *Gastroenterologie - Patologie, Dispozitive şi Tehnici Medicale, Simulare Clinică, Telemedicină* (Gastroenterology - Pathology, Devices and Medical Techniques, Clinical Simulation, Telemedicine) (2013), and co-authored *Curs intensiv de boli digestive* (Intensive Course of digestive diseases) (2013).

Ioana TODOR is currently a Lecturer at the University of Alba Iulia, Romania. She holds a BA in Psychology an MA in Psychological Counselling and Psychotherapy, and a PhD in Psychology from the "Babeş-Bolyai" University of Cluj-Napoca, Romania,. Her main research interests are cognitive inhibition and mental suppression of unwanted thoughts, social stigma associated with mental disorders, cognitive particularities in alcohol dependence and, generally speaking, and applications of cognitive psychology in education. She has authored *Uitarea intenţionată a stereotipurilor* (Intentional Forgetting of Stereotypes) (2013) and *Psihologie generală* (General Psychology) (2013).

Delia-Nicoleta TOMICI is currently a Social Work Assistant for the Caritas Federation, Timișoara, Romania. She holds a BA in Psychology from the "Tibiscus" University of Timişoara, Romania and an MA in Social Work from the West University of Timişoara. Her main research interests are psychological defence mechanisms and coping mechanisms in vulnerable groups.

Delia VÎRGĂ is currently an Associate Professor at the West University of Timișoara, Romania. She holds a BA in Psychology from the same University, and a PhD in Organizational Psychology from the "Babeş-Bolyai" University of Cluj-Napoca, Romania. Her main research interests are positive psychology applied in organizational life, how personal and job resources affect well-being and performance, work-family interaction, and work engagement and burnout. She has authored *Decizie și schimbare organizațională* (Decision and Organizational Change) (2007) and *Psihologie Experimentală—de la teorie la practică* (Experimental Psychology: From Theory to Practice) (2012).

Florentin VLAD is currently a Judge in Arad, Romania, and a PhD Candidate at the West University of Timişoara, Romania. He holds a BA in Law from the "Nicolae Titulescu" University of Craiova, Romania, and an MA in International Human Rights from the University of Bucharest, Romania. His main research interests are criminology, criminal law, and forensics. He has ublished widely in the field of law.